Awaken the Sexy Within

Awaken the SEXY WITHIN

Transform Your Body Fast with Your
Guaranteed Blueprint for Success

ROBB EVANS

NEW YORK

LONDON • NASHVILLE • MELBOURNE • VANCOUVER

Awaken the Sexy Within

Transform your Body Fast with your Guaranteed Blueprint to Success

Published in New York, New York, by Morgan James Publishing. Morgan James is a trademark of Morgan James, LLC. www.MorganJamesPublishing.com

ISBN 9781642797008 paperback
ISBN 9781642797015 eBook
Library of Congress Control Number: 2019944908

Cover Design by:
Megan Dillon
megan@creativeninjadesigns.com

Interior Design by:
Christopher Kirk
www.GFSstudio.com

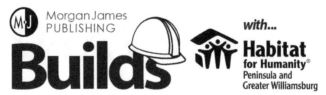

Morgan James is a proud partner of Habitat for Humanity Peninsula and Greater Williamsburg. Partners in building since 2006.

Get involved today! Visit
MorganJamesPublishing.com/giving-back

To Cherie, your unconditional love and support has inspired me
to transform lives through the power of sexiness.

To Emily and Olivia, you help me become a better Dad for you every day.

To those who want a healthier, stronger, fitter, and sexier versions of themselves.

Contents

Foreword

We are so connected in today's world. Everything we need is at our fingertips. The world really is our oyster. Just "google it" is a term used millions of times a day. If you want to lose weight—just "google it." If you're looking for a recipe—just "google it." If you want to get bigger biceps—just "google it!"

So, if it's all out there, why is the world still struggling with obesity and obesity-related diseases? Why do we suffer from self-image and self-confidence issues?

Much of the reason is that all the information on how to deal with these issues is scattered. It's all in bits and pieces, and if only one piece of the puzzle is addressed, then results won't happen.

So, when I first read Robb's book, I jumped for joy. Now, in one place, in order and made simple, step by step, you can 100% totally transform your body, your health, and your mindset.

There are so many books out there with exercises, recipes, and especially mindset but, until now, I have never found one that includes all this in ONE!

Robb has drawn from his own incredible story of being bullied and contemplating suicide as a young boy to now being an authority in health, fitness, nutrition, and body transformation. He has expertly pieced together the ultimate guide to help you find your sexy! To build, or get back, your best body, inside and out. To build or regain that confidence to look in the mirror and be happy with what you see.

Robb makes the process fun and simple. The mindset exercises are eye-opening and will really help guide you to creating the right thoughts, which create emotions that will lead to actions and eventually create your results.

This is a complete guide to body transformation. With 43 easy actionable steps to guide and produce guaranteed results, Robb has nailed the process. If you are willing, there is always a way. I know for a fact that without the right mindset, there's no way we would have succeeded in our sport. Mindset is everything, so make sure you do those parts of the process, as they are the key to success. Once your mindset is in check, everything else will seem easy.

The mindset guidance, the exercises you will go through, the recipes and workouts and the training calendars and templates to plan and organize it all are priceless and make for a clear pathway to realizing your health and wellness goals. Being healthy and happy IS sexy, so watch out—you may end up being in high demand!

Awaken the Sexy within will provide you with everything you need to completely transform your body and your mind and fit seamlessly into your everyday busy lifestyle.

Kerri Pottharst
Three-time Olympian gold medalist,
motivational speaker, mum, and
health and wellness advocate

Acknowledgements

I thank Cherie and my two daughters, Emily and Olivia, for believing in me and sacrificing their time with me while I focused on my mission. Your strength, unconditional love, and support have enabled me to dig a tunnel through the mountain and find the light at the end. I feel so blessed to have you in my life. I am a better partner, lover, coach, friend, Dad, and human being because of the impact you all have in inspiring me to grow.

I thank and acknowledge my coach, JT Foxx, the world's number-one wealth coach. You showed me the way to self-belief, hard work, focus, and the power of never giving in to excuses. You gave me the hunger to turn my vision into the reality of *Awaken the Sexy within*. I thank you for the incredible opportunities you have created for me to meet the most amazing people in the world. JT remains the clearest and most compelling voice in wealth creation and has changed the world of coaching forever.

I thank my late Mom and Dad for giving me life and showing me the power and depth of loving relationships. I thank my Mom for giving me the writing bug and the joy that books bring to your life. Mom showed me that anything is possible if you put your mind to it. Dad taught me the value of patience and practice to create perfection.

Thank you to Jeff Lazarus, my guardian angel, who has guided me through the maze from manuscript to published *Awaken the Sexy within*. You are the gift that keeps on giving, and your knowledge and support throughout have been incredible. Thank you, Jeff, for your friendship, spirit, and passion. You have helped me bring my words to life, enabling them to be shared with others around the world.

Emilie Bingham, my editor, was introduced to me by Jeff Lazarus. Words are not just words, and you have an incredible gift to reshape them to have a deeper and more meaningful impact. Thank you, Emilie; I am so grateful for your artistry.

Thank you to Nikki Sakavicius and Dann Thomas for spending tireless hours taking photos and producing beautifully presented images and video for me. *Awaken the Sexy within* would not be complete without your commitment and dedication. Thank you.

Thank you to David Hancock, founder of Morgan James Publishing, and his incredible team for believing in my vision and taking it to the people. I am so grateful to you.

Finally, I thank all of those who have supported my programs and training over the past decade. It has meant so much to me to see your transformations and hear how you are now living life on a higher level.

Introduction

I 'd like to take you on a brief journey into my life. I want you to see how I have taken my life from the lowest of lows to the highest of highs with my mind and body.

Today, I run a successful fitness business helping people globally. It's my passion, and I don't feel like I've worked a day in my life because of that passion. I have the most incredible relationships with the most amazing people around the world and love my life immensely.

But it wasn't always that way. Let's go back to the beginning. I grew up in Bendigo, Central Victoria, Australia, and from the age of 11, you could say I knew I was different. I was the shortest person in my school, had permed blonde hair and a dark birthmark on my face, played the bagpipes, and regularly wore a kilt. As I write this, I'm trying to convince myself that this *was* the trend at the time!

You see, at the time, it felt like I had no other talent. I was too small for football or cricket, couldn't swim, wasn't fast enough to run competitively. I never got picked to play in the school teams, so I turned to the bagpipes. I competed in competitions all around the state and won more times than I lost. I had found something that I was good at.

School was hard work for me, and I struggled through my classes. I didn't enjoy it, and, maybe thanks to the bagpipes, I didn't have many friends. On top of that, I remained the smallest person in school until I was 14 years old, making me an easy target for bullies. It wasn't uncommon to see me being pushed over and dragged down the long corridors by my feet by a couple of bigger kids. Lacking the confidence to speak up or lash out, I just kept putting up with it. I wouldn't say it was a daily occurrence, but over time, these attacks really damaged my self-image, my self-confidence, and my perception of self-worth.

Nowadays, we talk to our kids about bullying and how to speak up when they're in trouble. Back then, I don't recall thinking I shouldn't say anything to a teacher or my parents, but I didn't. I internalized it all instead.

An Ending before the Beginning

Sometimes you can only take so much for so long.

After years of being picked on for my size, for the way I looked, for the hobbies I took part in, I had had enough. One day, after a particularly bad day at school, I went to my room, closed the door, and just felt sad. Overwhelmingly sad. I didn't know how to change what I was feeling, and I was tired of it.

Part of the traditional Scottish battle dress was something we call a *skhi-undhu*, a small knife that was worn in your sock when you are on parade. I used to keep it in the bottom of a chest of drawers in my wardrobe. I went over to the drawer, took the knife out, and looked at it for a while. I just wanted to be happy. I wanted my life to be different. After a few moments, I took the skhi-undhu out of its sheath. Slowly, I raised the knife to my throat with both hands. I closed my eyes and thought about all the reasons I wanted it to end. All I knew in that moment was that I didn't want to keep feeling the same way anymore. Life felt cruel. I didn't know how to change that. I couldn't see a way out.

Something happened in the next 30 seconds. I froze. Part of me wanted to end it, but part of me knew this was just the beginning. I was 13 years old, and though I was in a world of hurt, I didn't know where life would take me. I didn't know if things would get better.

And yet, a little voice inside me said that this wasn't what my life was about. I didn't know what it was about at the time, but I knew I had to try getting to a happier place. I put the knife away and decided that tomorrow was another day. I was still overwhelmingly sad, but I chose to keep putting one foot in front of the other in the hope that I would end up in a happy place one day.

Even as I write and relive my story here, it breaks my heart. I have two beautiful children, and the thought of them in a similar situation is painful. My sadness deepens even further when I realize now that no one reached out to me. Not one person around me noticed that I was in so much pain. I thought my pain was obvious, and so it seemed to me that no one cared. You could say that I felt helpless but hopeful of the unknown.

Perhaps I grew up in a time when the term *bully* was not something that was discussed openly. I felt that I had to deal with these things myself. I don't consciously remember thinking that I shouldn't tell my parents, but I didn't feel like they could help. I figured that I was the one that needed to change if I wanted things to be different.

Beyond this moment, I continued to struggle on through school. By year 10, the bullying mostly stopped (I found a much taller friend to hang out with), but my self-confidence was still not good. The pressure mounted to pick an area of study to focus on, and I didn't know what I wanted. I wasn't great at many subjects, but I was decent at math and liked the exactness of the numbers.

Over the next 2 years, I went on to study accounting and business subjects and figured that I may as well complete a university degree, a bachelor of business in accounting. Back in the early '90s, there were plenty of accounting jobs around, and it seemed like a great way to make a good income and maybe start to feel better about my place in the world.

The Day I Chose to Begin My "Sexiness Journey"

At university one day, I was sitting in a behavioral science class. We had an individual in the class who had a habit of saying things that were off topic. It was disruptive but, at times, amusing. This day, he said something that made me laugh, and I had trouble containing myself. He glared at me across the classroom, and at the end of the class—in front of everyone—he ran at me from the other side of the room. He grabbed the table I was sitting at, pushed it into my stomach and rammed me up against the wall, threatening to kill me the whole time. Amazingly, the teacher didn't say anything. No one in the class said anything, and none of my friends came to help. I felt embarrassed and, because no one stood up for me, like it was my fault. Like I had brought this on because I didn't know how to talk to people.

I had flashes back to my childhood and to that afternoon with the skhi-undhu. I felt all the same self-doubt and insecurity that had led me to that point. But then I thought, *I'm getting too old for this!*

I needed to make a change. I was so sick and tired of feeling this way. That day was the day I decided to change my life. Never again was I going to feel helpless and sorry for myself. I'd had enough.

And the way I was going to do this was by changing my body.

A few days before, I had picked up the local paper and read an article about a young man who had put on 22 pounds (10 kilograms) of muscle in 10 weeks at a local gym. Reading it, I felt inspired to achieve something for myself. I wanted to undertake a complete metamorphosis that would make people say "Wow! Have you been working out?" I said to myself, *That's what I'm going to do!*

When I look back, I can see that in that moment, nothing had really changed in who I was. I was still the same person. Why was I inspired now to change my body? The answer is easy. I was tired of people treating me badly. I thought that if I were bigger and more in shape, I may have an easier time fitting in. The word that kept repeating in my mind was *sexy*. I wanted to be seen as sexy. But the very least, I wanted to defend myself if anyone ever physically went after me again.

So I drove out to the gym I'd been reading about and met with the owner. I told him what I wanted to do, that my goal was to grow out of every item of clothing I owned, down to my underwear. Fortunately, the gym owner, Laurie, was an ex-Olympic lifter, power lifter, and bodybuilder. I remember he put me on the scales fully clothed, and I weighed in at 110 pounds (50 kilograms).

"Wow. There's not much of you, is there?" he said.

To which I replied, "That's why I'm here, Laurie—to change all of that!"

Well, guess what? In 10 weeks, I put on that 22 pounds (10 kilograms) of muscle. I had done it. I had grown out of every pair of my wardrobe and every pair of underwear I owned. A very proud moment indeed.

More than that, I felt good about myself. It was the first sign of self-confidence for me. Until this point, I had felt like my height, weight, and appearance had controlled my life and how I related to other people. Learning to control what I could about my appearance felt like I was also gaining control over my place in the world and how people viewed me. This was in 1988. And from then on, heath, fitness, and nutrition have become integral parts of my life.

But I still had more to learn.

What Sexiness Really Means

As I mentioned, I was pretty good at math in school. After graduation, I kept with it and took a job at a large accounting firm in Melbourne. But after only a few years, I grew bored. To switch things up, I left that firm and joined the Royal Automobile Club of Victoria (RACV), where, luckily, there was such a wide array of jobs that I was able to continue switching it up every few years, working my way up the corporate ladder while also avoiding boredom.

But after 13 years of ladder climbing at RACV, I still couldn't honestly say that I *loved* my job. You know that feeling people describe when they say they don't feel like they work because they love what they do so much? I wanted to feel like that.

One day, I was working out in my regular gym. I'm not a religious person, but I am spiritual and like to think of my gym as being like my church. I feel at peace there and have had many creative moments in that environment. This day, I was racking my brain over what I could do with the rest of my working life. I was sitting on the edge of my bench press when I looked up at the ceiling and felt like a massive light bulb switched on.

I thought, *Why don't I just do this—become a fitness coach?*

It was like everything clicked into place in that moment. The idea of teaching others to achieve their fitness goals felt right.

More than that, I felt like I could do more than teach them how to lose weight or build up muscle. Around that time, I had a realization about my own fitness journey. For many years, I had maintained a healthy lifestyle and saw my body change and strengthen. The motivation had always been to fit in better with others—to prove my own worth to them. But after years of bullying, I had a hard time believing in myself.

I picked over my appearance in the mirror when my confidence was low. I took rudeness from others very personally. I had made over my body, but I hadn't finished making over my mind. So I set a new goal for myself: to feel good about my body naked.

I wanted to stand in front of the mirror with no clothes on and feel completely comfortable with myself. I wanted to know that I had worked hard and done everything I could at the gym to make my body strong and healthy. I wanted to see the food that I put into my body reflected in my muscles.

I knew I could never change my height, and so I couldn't compare myself to anyone but the man I had been the day before. My goal was no longer to look good for other people but to look good for myself. To see health reflected in the person in the mirror and to feel comfortable with that guy.

Decades after making a decision to become "sexy," I learned what true sexiness really was.

I went home that evening and talked the idea over with my wife at the time and committed to getting my fitness qualifications. It was a win–win. I could do more of what I loved, and my wife and I could spend more time together with our kids.

In 2009, I left the corporate world and launched Studioz Personal Training and Pakenham Boot Camps for Women. My first client was an employee at RACV, who lost 22 pounds (10 kilograms) in the 6 weeks we worked together.

Today, our business has worked with thousands of people wanting to improve their health and fitness. All shapes, all sizes, all ages. Men, women, and children of all levels of fitness. We have helped everyone from professional, world-class athletes to 11-year-old children being bullied at school.

We've helped our clients lose over 11,000 pounds (5,000 kilograms) of fat.

And we've donated more than $250,000 in services to local charities, community services, schools, kindergartens, and sporting clubs. We created a free nutrition program for children called Kids Munch It (www.KidsMunchIt.com.au) and have helped over 500 children learn more about how and why to eat well.

We launched our podcast www.RobbEvans365.com in 2018 to help people all over the world optimize their health and find their sexiness. And we have a lot more coming, including our online courses.

But what matters most is that I've changed my life. I know what I am meant to do. My purpose is to help others transform their lives and become the ultimate person that they've dreamed about becoming. It is to empower, motivate, inspire, and educate them. It's an incredibly rewarding job, and I *love* it.

When I was 13 years old and in a world of sadness, I could never have imagined I would be where I am today, helping people around the globe to feel good about themselves. This career has truly awoken an energy and passion inside me that makes me feel unstoppable. It nurtures me in a way that I can only liken to releasing endorphins for my soul. It allows me to be the true and best version of myself. I thrive from every pore as a result. It's a beautiful gift.

And it is one that you simply must experience for yourself.

Now it's your turn. This book asks you to take massive action to change your life forever. This book is about awakening the sexiness within yourself, achieving a physical transformation and about seeing yourself in the mirror and feeling *good* about the person looking back. I will show you how to achieve it, but it's you who must take the massive (that's right, massive) action to achieve it.

Everyone has their own journey in life. You've read a little about mine. It's time for you to embark on a new one—a body transformation journey.

To your sexiness,
ROBB EVANS

CHAPTER 1

Plan to Be Sexy; Never Fail to Plan

Winston Churchill once said, "He who fails to plan is planning to fail." This is critical to remember when you set out on your body transformation journey. I'm a huge fan of acting fast when you've decided on and committed to a fitness regime, but most people simply start without any plan as to how they'll maintain that regime beyond the first 14 days. And when results don't show up immediately, they're discouraged and jump into the next thing they think will work better. To this, I have one thing to say: Don't be like that!

Over the past decade, I've worked with thousands of clients. In doing so, I have tested and refined this program and the workouts to be fun, focused, and (most importantly) results driven. The bottom line is if you follow the program I've outlined for you, transformation will follow. You may be surprised to learn that achieving a body transformation does not require huge effort at every workout. What it does require is small, consistent action taken daily. Talk to any of my clients who have either reached their transformation goal or are on the way to achieving it, and they will tell you that they didn't make any hugely significant lifestyle changes to achieve the results. They will all agree that it was small

9

changes that they've made and implemented them every single day. That's right, every single day!

Body transformation is not a magic pill. Rather, it's a science. Right here, in this book, I'm giving you the scientific approach to achieving your very own transformation. This program works every time and achieves outstanding, life-sustainable change.

But there's a catch.

As foolproof as this program is, it will *not* help you achieve transformation by sitting on the shelf. Do the work; get the results. I'll teach you the rest, but right now you need to commit and resolve to completely transform your body forever. Not just for an upcoming event like a wedding or a beach vacation. But for the rest of your life.

I've been implementing the science I'm about to teach you for over 30 years, and the more I've learned, the more I've refined my approach. In *Awaken the Sexy within*, there are no diets, expensive equipment, or gym memberships required to achieve your body transformation. Only innovative, fun, safe, and sustainable techniques that can be easily integrated into your life.

And a plan.

Creating Your Plan

Let me ask you a question. If you were planning a road trip across the country, would you just jump in the car and start driving? I'm pretty sure most of you would say no. You must make plans for someone to look after the house while you're away, get the car serviced, decide where to stay each night, figure out the quickest route, make a playlist, stop for snacks, pack clothes, get gas. There's quite a lot of planning that needs to take place before you hit the road.

Your body transformation journey is no different. The difficulty is that most people do just start exercising or following a crash diet without first planning. Whether you've done it or know someone who has, I'm sure you've heard stories of people who lose 22 pounds (10 kilograms) only to put all that weight back on, plus more. I guarantee that those who have experienced this phenomenon didn't have a clearly articulated plan that empowered them to make sustainable change.

Before we move on to writing down your plan for success, I need you to read this next sentence very carefully.

WARNING!
You are not to move on in this book until you complete
each action item before you. It is a crucial element
to your success and cannot be skipped for any reason.

ACTION 1: THE NAKED TRUTH

Stand in front of the mirror for the next step. Remove all your clothes and stand facing the mirror. Look at each part of your body, from head to toe. Look at the features you like, and notice why that is. Look at the parts you find less flattering, and notice what you would like to improve. How would you describe what you are seeing? Do this same exercise when you turn to the right; then turn to the right again, and look over your shoulder at your back, legs, and bottom; turn to the right again, and look at the other side. Take a few minutes to write down your responses to what you've seen. Be as specific and detailed as possible.

_____

_____

_____

_____

_____

_____

_____

ACTION 2: THE SELF-ANALYSIS

Write down what you liked and why. Be sure to use emotive language to describe your feelings. Write down what you didn't like and why. Again, be sure to use emotive language.

_____

_____

_____

_____

_____

_____

ACTION 3: HOW SEXY DO YOU FEEL?

In this moment, how would you rate your perception of your own sexiness out of 10, with 10 being 100% supreme sexiness, Adonis or goddess, and 0 being disgusted with yourself.

_____

_____

_____

_____

My Self-Perception

Sexiness has many different meanings to people. In a moment, I'm going to ask you to define the meaning of sexiness to you. Before I do that, I will give you my meaning of sexiness. When I was a teenager, I had a horrible self-image. I was short, small-framed, skinny, and not muscular; I thought I was ugly because I didn't like my hair; I had a chipped front tooth and an ugly birthmark on my face the size of your thumb. I hated my body!

As I became an adult, I still didn't think I was sexy at all. At the time, I felt I needed to be taller, to be more muscular, to have better teeth, to have no blemishes on my face, to have hair like a model and a great personality. For many years, I struggled with my self-image because I felt I had no control over my size, my teeth, my face, or my hair, so I just had to settle. As stupid as it sounds, it was my reality.

I have mentioned before that it's not possible to control all the things that happen in your life. I couldn't be taller; my face, teeth, and hair were given to me this way without my control. You could suggest that I have surgery and hairstyling in these areas and I could change them. But those options can only do so much and weren't options for me. Plus, they wouldn't have fixed the inner version of me. The reality was that the inner version of myself was ugly, not the outside. I can't control those other aspects of my life. But I can always control what everything in my life means to me. After many years of self-reflection, I realized that I needed to work hard on my body to achieve the look I wanted, but I also needed to work hard on my self-talk.

Here is how I now define the qualities in me that make me sexy:

- I am equally as human as everyone else on this planet.
- I treat others the way I would like to be treated.
- My purpose in life is to serve others by educating, inspiring, and empowering them to transform their minds and bodies. I do this through helping them optimize their health with sustainable nutrition and exercise they can perform for the rest of their life.
- I am passionate and energized.
- I love passionately and deeply without limits.
- I am an amazing lover.

- I love myself for who I am, what I have done in the past, and who I am becoming.
- I work on my body every day to make myself the best possible version I can.
- My height, teeth, face, and hair are no longer important to me because I love myself the way I am.
- People who love me for who I am are the people I have—and want—in my life.
- I have a great personality and sense of humor that create a sexy aura.
- I work on improving my mind, body, and spirit every single day.
- I am sexy the way I am, but I want to look great naked, and I can be sexier!

Notice how my definition and meaning of sexiness changed. Initially, my definition only focused on the physical. My meaning now has more meaning attached to my mindset and who I am as a person and the qualities I bring to the world. It's taken many years for me to feel comfortable in my own skin. The great news is that I transformed my thinking as well as my body. If I can do it, so can you. I believe it's the ultimate beautiful gift that you can give to yourself.

Would you agree that it is possible that sexiness has absolutely nothing to do with your size? I believe the answer to that comes down to personal preference. Look at the voluptuous "models" that were depicted in ancient paintings. They weren't fit looking ladies. They were ladies that would be considered overweight by our measure of body mass index. At the time, they were revered by others, especially the poor. Being overweight was a social status symbol of significance and sexiness. Some cultures believe that a super skinny physique is sexy. Many in the Japanese culture find that sumo wrestlers are sexy. Many in Western cultures may not agree. There's no right or wrong. It is an individual choice.

My guess is that you've picked up this book because you want a higher level of sexiness in your life. That means you do want a greater outcome for yourself. More energy, more defined, lighter, less body fat, more muscular, more toned body, better arms, shoulders, chest legs, butt, back, and tummy. It may be a combination of some or all those features. The objective is to get your body and mindset in the right place for you to achieve the ultimate sexy you. You're getting all the essential tools in *Awaken the Sexy within* to transform your physical body and mind. I've provided a separate chapter here specifically on mindset sexiness because I know when I came to peace with who I was and what I wanted, my reasons became so much clearer. This then led to greater results and a dramatic increase in the way I viewed my sexiness. Not just how I perceived myself but how my partner perceived me too. Let me put it another way. Physical sexy is no good to you if you don't have mindset sexiness. Beautiful and sexy on the outside but ugly on the inside is a recipe for disaster.

I'm not suggesting that you need to be arrogant and a show-off about how you feel about yourself, but I am suggesting you strengthen the sexiness image you hold for yourself. Having this image of the ultimate you and the reasons for it will drive you. Trust me, if you have an intimate partner, it will drive them wild! You bring more sexiness and energy into the bedroom, and watch how your life starts to look better. At some level, we all want to feel sexy, desired, loved, and craved in a way that creates a molten fury of passion throughout our physiology, heart, and soul in a way that leaves you completely breathless.

ACTION 4: DEFINING YOUR SEXINESS

Write down how you would define sexiness in a way that is deeply meaningful and connecting to you. Remember, this is not about anyone else's influence of what is sexy but, rather, about how you define sexiness for yourself. Be very clear and specific about what you mean. Use emotive language that lights a fire within you. Don't be shy. No one else needs to read your definition. Imagine how amazing you will feel once you have met the terms of your definition.

Once you have done this, go back to action 3 and see whether it changes how you rate your current level of sexiness. Make a note of any changes and the reasons for them.

_____

_____

_____

_____

_____

_____

_____

_____

_____

Having completed those tasks, I know there will be some gaps between where you want to be and where you are in this moment. I want you to take some time now to think about those gaps between your definition of sexiness and how you could feel even sexier.

ACTION 5: HOW TO FEEL SEXIER

Write down at least three things you could change about your mindset to make you feel sexier and to help you meet your definition of sexiness.

_____

_____

_____

_____

_____

I believe in the power of incantations. An incantation is a phrase you say to yourself, out loud, with emotion and passion so that you feel it throughout your body and nervous system. It's not just thinking positively; it's a statement driven by a vision and belief system. For it to be effective, you must first write it down to be clear about what you will incant.

By way of example, I have used these phrases over time with great success. If you are thinking that this step is a little crazy, then have a little faith and trust the process. What I first thought was silly turned into be the greatest gift in reprogramming my mind:

- The power of sexiness is within me now.
- Every day, I'm becoming stronger, healthier, and the best version of me possible.
- My level of sexiness is controlled by my mind, body, and spirit.
- Every day I'm feeling more and more sexy.
- Age is no barrier to the level of sexiness I can achieve.
- You are sexy, and I love who you are.

The key with an incantation is to believe it's for you. Say it out loud, with so much passion and conviction that you believe you've already achieved it. That's why it is called an incantation! To be successful, you must incant these phrases over and over and over and over and over, every single day until they become a part of you. This may take days, weeks, or months. The point is not to stop until you reach your goal. Don't just say them in your head; say them out loud. In your car, while driving, in the shower, anywhere! I used to walk through the streets around my neighborhood, belting out my incantations, and I can tell you I would get some strange looks from people sometimes. But I didn't care. I knew my purpose. Don't let other people's judgments of you shake you from your path. I found a smile and a hello did wonders and probably gave them something to talk about later in the day.

ACTION 6: INCANT YOUR WAY TO EMPOWERMENT

Write down at least three variations of incantations you will use to help build your arsenal of tools to create your sexy image of yourself along with the sexy body you desire.

See if you can identify your phrase with a jingle or rhythm to make it flow nicely.

_____

_____

_____

_____

_____

_____

_____

ACTION 7: ACT NOW—INCANT!

Say these incantations at least 20 times per day out loud, stating with 100% emotion, belief, excitement, and passion. That means you need to be LOUD as your saying them!

WAIT! I can see that some of you are going to skip this step because you think it's not important. You might think, *No one has asked me to do this before, I've never done it before, I don't see how it relates to transforming me, it's not important, it's not going to work,* or *I don't need to do that to be successful.* I hear you and understand the reservations you may have. But you must understand that change is difficult, and to achieve the transformational change you want is most likely going to require an approach different from what you have undertaken in the past. I know this is different. But I also know the incredible power that it holds. You need to have faith in the process and feel me when I tell you this step has the potential to be life changing for you. Even if you don't believe me, do it anyway, and see for yourself!

You are well on the way to completely awaken your sexy.

ACTION 8: CREATING YOUR WHAT, WHY, COMMITMENT, AND MUSTS

Before we go any further, let's spend some time identifying why you want to achieve a body transformation. What is it that will drive you to keep going past the first few weeks? What does success look like for you? The answers to these questions are important for creating your personal plan to change your life.

I have provided you with some space here to write your answers, but I'm a wordy guy. I'd take out a note pad or open a fresh document on the computer and start writing. Don't think about your answers too hard. But spend the time to commit them to writing. It will slow your thinking down, reinforce your thoughts, and become an important reference to keep you focused.

Make sure you have at least 45 minutes of quiet time to give this exercise the attention it needs.

What You Want to Achieve

The Bible says, "Where there is no vision, people perish." Write down your vision for your health and fitness journey.

Describe in detail how you want to look and feel. Use empowering, emotive language that has deep meaning to you. There is no right or wrong here; just write it in a way that will drive you forward.

For example, here is my vision. (Keep in mind that this is simply what was right for me at the time of writing this.)

To look amazing naked! Have a physical body that I love with boundless energy, strength, and happiness that touches everyone I meet. I want to represent all that is possible and exciting about life.

_____

_____

_____

_____

Why You Want It

Now that you have created your vision, I want you to clearly—and powerfully—articulate why it is important for you to achieve it.

In creating your *why*, write down your responses to these questions:

- What will it mean when you accomplish your vision?
- What has stopped you in the past?
- Why will you make this time different?
- What will your body transformation mean for your relationships?
- What will it mean for your self-confidence and self-image?
- What will it mean for your career?
- What will it mean to your family, children, etc.?
- What will you do with a dramatic improvement in your energy?

_____

_____

_____

_____

Now, if you're up to this point and you haven't written down responses for each one of these questions, STOP! Go back and answer each question.

Do you think Olympic medalists like Kerri Pottharst accidentally won their gold medals? No, of course not. It took hard work, pain, setbacks, heartache, a detailed plan, and tons of focus. But they kept pushing through because their *why* for doing it had such deep meaning to them.

You need to create that hunger for yourself, which is why I've asked you to write your responses to the above questions. It channels your focus and energy into understanding why you *really* want your body transformation.

Considering everything you've just written down, create a powerful statement that explains why you will achieve your body transformation vision.

Go for it! Don't edit yourself; just write and write.

Here's mine:

To be the absolute best version of the physical me that I can be. I want to optimize my health; look sexy; be powerful, muscular, and strong; and have a limitless supply of energy to lead the life I want. I must have fun and enjoy the process. I want to be an amazing role model for my soul mate and children.

_____

_____

_____

_____

How Committed Are You to Achieving Your Body Transformation (from 0% to 100%)?

Change is difficult. You've got to fight through it and have a hunger for being successful. Your level of commitment will have a direct correlation to the outcome you achieve. If someone is only 10% committed, meaning they'll "give it a try," how likely do you think they are to succeed? I ask this question of all my clients, and I don't take on anyone that has a commitment level of less than 70%. I do this because I only want to work with people that are absolutely committed to change. If someone doesn't *really* want to change, they won't.

If your commitment level is less than 100%, be honest; write down at least three reasons for why that is.

If your commitment level is less than 100%, write down three actions you can take over the next 24 hours to increase your commitment level.

Why is your commitment less than 100%?

1. _____

2. _____

3. _____

What can you do to bring it up?

1. _____

2. _____

3. _____

Why you MUST make the change right now.

Still not at 100%? Let's finish this exercise up by writing down all the reasons you know you need to start this body transformation right now. Why is now the right time for you?

Then, write down everything you'll miss out on if you don't take advantage of this opportunity to transform your body. What will giving up cost you?

Write down seven reasons you absolutely must change right now to achieve your body transformation.

1. _____

2. _____

3. _____

4. _____

5. _____

6. _____

7. _____

Write down seven things it will cost you if you don't change right now.

1. _____

2. _____

3. _____

4. _____

5. _____

6. _____

7. _____

ACTION 9: SETTING YOUR GOALS

Success is a science. Find someone who has achieved amazing outcomes in the area that you want to become successful, and copy what they're doing. That is the fastest way to success. Lucky for you, that's me. I've helped my clients lose literally thousands of pounds of fat through the exact same strategies I'm outlining in this book. And I've learned that a key component of any successful journey is setting goals that are specifically meaningful and inspirational to you. They should be challenging goals that push you out of your comfort zone. Goals that stretch you, make you feel uncomfortable, and maybe even scare you.

Success will not show up by accident. Setting specific goals for your health and fitness is fundamental to your success. In the next exercise, write down the goals you would like to achieve over the next 12 months. Then I'd like you to break those goals down further into 12-week blocks.

We do this for a few reasons. First, it's important to know exactly what you are aiming for. However, if the goal feels too large, you may become immobilized by the fear. If you want to lose 110 pounds (50 kilograms), you can't focus on that number. Instead, break the number down into smaller goals, like 2.2 pounds (1 kilogram) per week. That's much more manageable and gives you a focus on a weekly basis. It may seem like an insignificant step, but each step is powerful.

Maybe you've tried and failed before? If so, did you do these exercises last time? If you've made it this far into *Awaken the Sexy within*, then you haven't failed. You only fail if you give up. Once again, trust me when I say that all my successful clients have had clearly articulated goals in their mind. You need to do the same.

Write down the body transformation goals you have for yourself over the next 12 months.

12-Month Body Transformation Goals

Quarterly Goals
January to March
April to June
July to September
October to December

DO NOT MOVE ON TO THE NEXT CHAPTER UNTIL YOU HAVE COMPLETED EVERY ACTION ITEM ABOVE. NO EXCUSES!

Summary

- You must have a plan. When you fail to plan, you plan to fail.
- You need to commit and resolve to completely transform your body forever. No one else can do that for you.
- Looking at yourself naked in the mirror is a powerful way to motivate you to act to change those parts of your body you would like to improve.

- Writing down how you feel about the current state of your body must involve emotive language to engage your neurological pathways with your physiology.
- Examining feelings around your current definition of sexiness will create a hunger for transformation.
- Creating a fun and playful name for your transformation journey will create energy and focus. For example, call your new self Energized Adonis, Sexy Kitty, Angel Warrior, etc.
- It is important to determine what you could change about your mindset to make you feel sexier to help you meet your definition of sexiness.
- Daily incantations are a great way to build your arsenal of tools to create your sexy self-image along with the sexy body you desire.
- Set goals that are specific and inspirational to you. Use these goals to push yourself out of your comfort zone.
- Everyone can awaken the sexy within.

SUCCESS STORY:
Ruth Eshuis, 27 years old

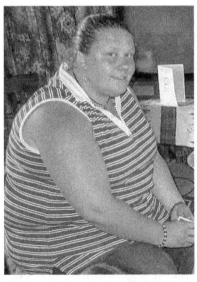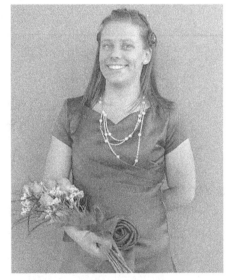

As you can see from the before and after photos, Ruth Eshuis has had the most amazing transformation. Ruth's before photo had her peaking at 297 pounds, and she is now an incredible 145 pounds lighter and has completely transformed her life. Ruth is such an inspiration to everyone that knows her. The photos say it all, but Ruth has lost in excess of 80 inches of fat from her chest, waist, hips, thighs, and arms. How did she do it? The key has been setting her up with a sustainable tailored meal plan based on the foods she likes and coaching her to embed a balanced resistance and cardio program that she can maintain forever.

"Becoming healthy has meant so much for me. I feel strong, well, freed, and equipped. I love my new routines and eating habits, and the fun of discovering many unexpected benefits of weight loss. What I've learned with Robb this year will help me for a lifetime, and it's even helped my family, friends, and coworkers to reach their fitness goals! Thanks, Robb."

CHAPTER 2

Eat Your Way to Sexiness

I want you to know that I have tremendous respect for you. You've taken the time to purchase a copy of *Awaken the Sexy within* because you want to make a change in yourself. You are different from most people, who accept where they are and aren't prepared to change. But not you. You want to be in the small percentage of people who achieve the body transformation they've always wanted. Congratulations!

Before we talk about fitness plans or specific workouts, we need to spend some time talking about food. I'm sure you already knew that transformation requires both activity and healthy eating. But your nutrition plays such a significant role in your transformation that, up to this point, the chances are high that you've been underestimating its importance. Is that fair to say? Can you honestly say that you've been honoring your body and fueling it in a way that enables you to perform at your highest level?

ACTION 10: YOUR CURRENT EATING HABITS

In order to establish a clear understanding of the kind of fuel you've been putting into your body, let's take these questions one step further. Write down in the space below everything you've eaten in the last 24 hours.

Meal Description	Additional Information
Breakfast: (Time:_____)	How much water did you drink? How many cups of tea? How many cups of water? How many soft drinks? How much alcohol?
AM Snack: (Time: _____)	Did you exercise? If so, for how long? How much sleep did you get last night?
Lunch: (Time: _____)	
PM Snack: (Time: _____)	
Dinner: (Time: _____)	
Evening Snack: (Time: _____)	

How did it go? Based on my experience, people will understate what they eat and overstate the amount of exercise they do by 10%–30%. The point of this exercise is not for you to beat yourself up because of what you are doing or not doing but, rather, for you to recognize your current habits with complete honesty.

Every day, I talk to people of all ages, sizes, demographics, and socioeconomic positions about food, exercise, and transformation. So many people tell me that their eating habits are fine and that all they need is someone to kick their butt with exercise. My response to that is usually something like, "You don't know what you don't know when it comes to your nutrition." Eating a salad for lunch, for example, does not mean that we can eat whatever we want the rest of the day. We may think we know what we're doing, but I've found that many people are just guessing. We have so many different food options presented to us that it's difficult to make sense of it all sometimes.

Of course, the marketing messages we are bombarded with every hour of the day don't help. Food manufacturers pay millions of dollars to marketers to sell their product. They are paid to come up with visually appealing products using the most powerful key words on their labels to connect with the most people. What that means is that just because a product sounds healthy, it doesn't mean it is. Low-fat, organic, low-calorie, low-carb, high-protein, low-sugar, all-natural, high in omega-3s, high fiber—these are all words they use to make us feel good about eating their foods. With so many choices, how do you know what's healthy and what's hype?

Diets Do Not Work

Before we go any farther, let's get one thing out of the way. There are many approaches to eating healthy and hundreds of diet plans that claim to be the only one worth following. However, while many of these approaches may make you feel better in the short-term, few give you a long-term transformation.

Long story short: I don't believe in diets. They're simply not sustainable.

My definition of success around nutrition is creating life-sustaining meal plans that include healthy, nutritious food with balanced levels of fiber, protein, good fats, low energy, and high energy. To determine if a diet plan is right for you, ask yourself, "Does it make sense to follow this diet for the rest of my life?"

If you can't follow it forever, I'd argue that it's not optimizing your health. If it's not optimizing your health, it's not worth your time. When I choose to work with a client, my goal is to optimize the entire person's health and mindset. I'm teaching them the exercise, nutrition, and lifestyle principles that they will live by from that point forward. My passion with nutrition is to educate people to make better choices. It's not rocket science, but it is a science.

WARNING!
YOU MUST READ THIS BEFORE YOU MAKE
ANY CHANGES TO YOUR DAILY NUTRITION

We're about to head into my principles of nutrition.
They are based on decades of research and training.
However, I don't know you personally.
I don't know your medical history, allergies,
food intolerances, eating preferences, etc.

I recommend seeking medical advice from your doctorbefore you make any changes to your daily nutrition plan. Show them your plan and include the sample meal plan provided next. You should make the necessary modifications to the plan with your doctor's guidance.

Energy In versus Energy Out

If you have been on a weight loss journey before or have done some research into the most effective strategies to lose weight, you will have come across the term *calories*. Even if you haven't, you've probably seen it on the nutrition labels on nearly every food. But there's confusion over what a calorie really is. Let me give you a brief overview in plain English.

A calorie is the amount of energy that is in the food. All foods have calories, and all of us need to consume a certain number of calories each day to maintain our constant body weight. This is what we call *energy in*.

We burn off calories when we are asleep and our bodily organs function to keep us alive and the blood circulating. This is called our basal metabolic rate. We also burn off more calories as we move each day, whether that be walking, cycling, or simply carrying heavy grocery bags. We gain weight when the energy coming in is higher than the energy going out.

It's a pretty simple concept; consume more than you burn off, and you will gain fat!

Let's take the example of an average middle-aged female weighing between 130 pounds (60 kilograms) and 175 pounds (80 kilograms). She would need to consume approximately 1600–1800 calories per day to maintain her current body weight. Now, this is a very simple example and doesn't consider body composition (percentage of body fat versus muscle and fluid), her activity levels, medical history, or height. However, logic tells you that if she needs 1600 calories to maintain her weight, simply eating less than that will cause weight loss. Although the mathematics is technically correct, it is not as simple as this.

If she ate 1200 calories across two meals each day, would that work as effectively as 1200 calories across three, four, five, or six meals per day? What if she cut her intake down to 900 calories per day? Would that work faster?

All good questions. The reality is that simply cutting calories can be a losing game. Proper consideration must be given to the foods that are being eaten, the frequency of meals, the size of the meals, and how the consumption of those meals impacts your metabolism. I've worked with many clients that have restricted their caloric intake for years and have not been able to successfully lose weight. Yet when we alter the types of foods they are eating, usually increasing the volume of food and the meal frequency to six times per day without increasing the calories, they often see instantaneous results. Why would that be the case? Because when the body becomes accustomed to a reduced caloric intake, it can go into starvation mode and slow your metabolism dramatically to cling onto any food that it does get. This can be very frustrating to many people and can make them lose faith in the possibility of a transformation.

Becoming Calorie Aware

Go to Google and type in *calorie calculator*. You will find several easy-to-use tools where you can enter your details and it will give you an approximate number of calories you should eat per day. Even though I create many meal plans where calories are not the focus, I do believe that following a calorie-controlled plan will certainly help you stay accountable for at least the first 12 weeks of your body transformation journey. You don't have to count the calories, but I strongly believe in being calorie aware. There's a big difference. Counting calories is very specific, requiring you to keep detailed accounts of everything you eat and their caloric value. However, if you follow the measurements I've outlined in the plans, you don't need to worry about counting the calories. The measurements take care of that for you.

For example, a simple milkshake could have more than 1000 calories in one glass! That's a lot, especially given that many meal plans I create for weight loss clients contain 1200–1500 calories for the entire day. If we look at vegetables by comparison, 1000 calories in vegetables would equate to five or six large dinner plates full of food, as well as a lean piece of chicken breast and ½ cup of brown rice. It's a huge amount of food that you wouldn't be able to eat in one sitting. Yet the milkshake is easily consumed and will probably still leave you unfulfilled. This is a drastic example, but when you become aware of these differences in calories, you won't have to count the calories—ever. You simply get a feel for the portion sizes and ingredients to assess whether it is high or low calorie.

As you travel along your journey, I encourage you to start to take initiative to further educate yourself about food. Grab food out of your pantry, and review the nutrition label. Look at the calories. Look at the other elements as well—fat, saturated, trans, proteins, carbs, sugars. Compare products that you would consider "sometimes" foods with something more nutritious and healthier. Take note of the various elements and what stands out to you. I always look at the calories first then move down the label from there. I don't expect you to understand every aspect of nutrition labels immediately, but as you educate yourself by comparing products and checking calories, protein, carbohydrate, and fat levels along with ingredient lists, you become empowered to know exactly what you are eating.

Natural Metabolic Boosters to Shape Your Sexiness

When I'm talking to clients about metabolism, I liken it to a car engine. The faster the metabolism, the faster you will burn fat from your body. There are several metabolic boosters you can naturally engage to speed up your results. For instance, the resistance training and cardiovascular exercise you perform can permanently increase your metabolism. This chapter is about nutrition, so I want to give you an incredible tip to increase your metabolism through the food that you eat. The more low-energy, plant-based food you eat, the faster your metabolism will be.

Most people do not follow the *Australian Dietary Guidelines* for eating fruit and vegetables (see https://www.eatforhealth.gov.au/guidelines/australian-guide-healthy-eating). The guidelines recommend at least five to six servings of vegetables and two servings of fruit per day for adults. Be honest with yourself right now and see if you eat enough fruit and vegetables. Most people eat enough fruit but struggle with the vegetables. The biggest serving of vegetables typically comes with the evening meal, but the rest of the day suffers.

Let's talk about how to fix that. I advise people to always eat plant-based foods that are colorful and crunchy, like carrots. The colorful part of our fruit and vegetables is important, because those foods are flooded with antioxidants and nutrients. The crunchy part of those foods is also very important. Think about this: Water, when you drink it, passes through your system quickly, and your body doesn't have to work very hard to process it. Now think about a carrot. First, you need to crunch it up in your mouth before swallowing. Once swallowed, the food sits in your stomach, waiting to be processed. Because the food is crunchy, your body must work hard to break it down, take up the nutrients, and eliminate the waste. Guess what that means? Your metabolism gets fired up to work hard in the process.

If you think this type of food sounds boring, then you're in for a surprise. All the meals included in the meal plans taste delicious and are suitable for the whole family. You don't have to be a chef, because, trust me, I'm not. They're easy for anyone to prepare.

It might seem obvious that you need to eat more of these plant-based foods, but you probably didn't know the powerful impact consuming these foods has on your metabolism. On top of all the improved health opportunities from eating fruit and vegetables, don't underestimate the amazing boost it gives to your fat-burning potential.

ACTION 11: FIND OPPORTUNITIES FOR IMPROVEMENT

Based on what you already know, write down the various improvement opportunities you can identify from what you wrote down in action 10. One of the best ways to learn is to write down your thoughts. I want you to use your existing skills to see how you would improve your own eating. When we get to the meal plans shortly, you can compare what you have written down below to the meal plans and see where there are differences. Some concepts may be revision or reaffirming what you already know; others may be brand new and "aha!" moments that can really shift you to another level.

Consider the following when writing down your list:

- Am I skipping meals?
- Am I eating snacks?
- Am I eating healthy and nutritious snacks?
- Are my food portions appropriate for my health and fitness goals?
- Am I drinking 50 ounces (1.5 liters) of water per day or more?
- Am I drinking too much coffee, tea, soft drinks, alcohol, fruit juice, etc.?
- Am I eating enough fruit and vegetables?
- Am I overindulging in fast food or takeout?
- Am I prepared for my meals, or are they always last minute or purchased meals?

_____

_____

_____

_____

_____

_____

_____

_____

_____

_____

Time to Eat!

I know you're eager to get to the heart of the matter. You're probably thinking, "Robb, just tell me what to eat!"

Well, here we go. Below, I've included some crucial nutrition principles that you can follow to optimize your health for the rest of your life. Keeping in mind that I could produce an entire book solely about nutrition, I thought it would be useful to not only provide you with generic principles but also to give you some specific examples of meal plans that I have prepared for clients who had tremendous transformational success.

Remember that these meal plans have been prepared for clients under my direct supervision, and it was safe for them to be placed on a 1200-calorie meal plan to assist them in losing fat, in conjunction with their tailored resistance and cardio training programs. 1200 calories may or may not be appropriate for you after discussions with your doctor or medical health professional who knows your health history.

Daily Nutrition Principles to Optimize Your Health

The following are some everyday keys to ensure you optimize your health through nutrition:

1. Consume six meals per day to help keep your metabolism rate high. Breakfast, lunch, and dinner, along with a morning snack, an afternoon snack, and an evening snack. My recommendation is that you consume a meal every 2–3 hours once you've had your breakfast.

2. A typical daily menu should contain the following:

   Breakfast: Protein in the form of egg whites, a protein drink, or low-fat yogurt + some plant-based food (e.g., fruits or vegetables) + some high-energy food (e.g., 1 cup of nutritious breakfast cereal or a piece of whole-wheat toast).

   Morning Snack: A small tub of low-fat, low-sugar yogurt or a piece of fruit.

   Lunch: Protein in the form of chicken, salmon, or tuna (approximately 4 ounces) + a salad mix with lots of color and crunch. Or one round of sandwiches on whole-wheat bread or one wrap filled with 4 ounces of protein and lots of salad.

   Afternoon Snack: Same as for morning snack.

   Dinner: Protein in the form of chicken, beef, fish, steak, or pork (approximately 4 ounces) + 3 cups of mixed colorful and crunchy vegetables + up to 1 cup of high-energy food, such as cooked brown rice, pasta, or sweet potato.

   Evening Snack: Popcorn (0.7 ounces), 2–4 small wheat crackers with some peanut butter or avocado or a piece of fruit and some low-fat, low-sugar yogurt.

3. Drink 50+ fluid ounces of water every day.

4. Aim for 6 hours of sleep per night to help keep you energized.

Below are several examples of different meal plans. What is important to remember is that these are designed as examples of meal portion size and their ingredients so that you can learn the principles of healthy eating. The ingredients change, but the principles stay the same. Why are the principles important? Because they provide the makeup of each component of the plan and true success comes from embedding these principles in your life forever.

That's right—forever!

Table 2.1. 1200-Calorie, No-Intolerances Meal Plan, Example 1

QTY	Measure	Description	Protein (g)	Carbs (g)	Fats (g)	Calories
Breakfast						
1	cup	Nonfat skim milk	8.40	11.90	0.40	86.00
0.5	cup	Egg whites	15.75	1.35	0.00	76.50
1	cup	Mixed vegetables	1.10	3.10	0.22	24.30
1	bag	Oatmeal (packet)	3.90	24.30	2.70	144.00
		Totals	**29.15**	**40.65**	**3.32**	**330.80**
AM Snack						
1	each	Apple	0.30	21.00	0.50	81.00
		Totals	**0.30**	**21.00**	**0.50**	**81.00**
Lunch						
4	oz	Chicken breast	23.00	0.00	1.60	110.00
0.4	oz	Croutons	1.00	6.40	1.80	46.50
1	tbsp	Reduced fat, Italian salad dressing	0.00	1.10	0.00	6.00
1	large	Mixed garden salad	2.60	19.00	0.80	98.00
		Totals	**26.60**	**26.50**	**4.20**	**260.50**
PM Snack						
1	cup	Nonfat yogurt	7.00	11.00	0.00	70.00
		Totals	**7.00**	**11.00**	**0.00**	**70.00**
Dinner						
0.5	cup	Brown rice, cooked	2.45	24.85	0.60	116.00
1	each	Chicken stir fry supreme*	30.38	11.38	4.21	240.11
		Totals	**32.83**	**36.23**	**4.81**	**356.11**
Evening Snack						
1	tbsp	Peanut butter	4.00	3.50	8.15	95.00
4	each	Wheat crackers	2.80	15.20	1.60	96.00
		Totals	**6.80**	**18.70**	**9.75**	**191.00**
Actual Totals			**102.68**	**154.08**	**22.58**	**1289.41**
Actual Percentage of Total Calories			**33.38**	**50.10**	**16.52**	**100.00**

* See the Recipes section for ingredients and cooking instructions.

Table 2.2. 1200-Calorie, No-Intolerances Meal Plan, Example 2

QTY	Measure	Description	Protein (g)	Carbs (g)	Fats (g)	Calories
Breakfast						
1.5	cup	Cheerios breakfast cereal	4.50	34.50	3.00	165.00
1	cup	Nonfat skim milk	8.40	11.90	0.40	86.00
1	cup	Strawberries	1.00	9.00	0.00	60.00
		Totals	**13.90**	**55.40**	**3.40**	**311.00**
AM Snack						
1	each	Apple	0.30	21.00	0.50	81.00
		Totals	**0.30**	**21.00**	**0.50**	**81.00**
Lunch						
1	each	Egg (whole, incl. yolk)	6.70	1.30	7.30	100.00
0.4	oz	Croutons	1.00	6.40	1.80	46.50
1	tbsp	Reduced-fat Italian salad dressing	0.00	1.10	0.00	6.00
1	large	Mixed garden salad	2.60	19.00	0.80	98.00
		Totals	**10.30**	**27.80**	**9.90**	**250.50**
PM Snack						
1	each	Carrot, raw, medium, cut into sticks	0.70	7.30	0.10	31.00
0.5	cup	Cottage cheese, 1% fat	14.00	3.10	1.15	82.00
		Totals	**14.70**	**10.40**	**1.25**	**113.00**
Dinner						
4	oz	Ribeye steak, grilled, lean	31.40	0.00	6.00	180.45
1	tbsp	Reduced-fat sour cream	0.44	0.64	1.80	20.25
3	cup	Mixed vegetables	3.30	9.30	0.66	72.90
5	tsp	Chunky salsa	0.00	7.50	0.00	25.00
4	oz	Potato	3.00	25.00	0.00	107.00
		Totals	**38.14**	**42.44**	**8.46**	**405.60**
Evening Snack						
1	each	Nonfat yogurt	7.00	11.00	0.00	70.00
		Totals	**7.00**	**11.00**	**0.00**	**70.00**
Actual Totals			**84.34**	**168.04**	**23.51**	**1231.10**
Actual Percentage of Total Calories			**27.63**	**55.04**	**17.33**	**100.00**

Table 2.3. 1200-Calorie, Gluten-Free Meal Plan, Example 1

QTY	Measure	Description	Protein (g)	Carbs (g)	Fats (g)	Calories
Breakfast						
1	each	Banana, medium	1.20	26.70	0.60	105.00
1	oz	Cereal	1.62	22.68	0.45	105.60
1	cup	Nonfat skim Milk	8.40	11.90	0.40	86.00
		Totals	**11.22**	**61.28**	**1.45**	**296.60**
AM Snack						
2	each	Mandarin	1.00	11.00	0.20	56.00
		Totals	**1.00**	**11.00**	**0.20**	**56.00**
Lunch						
0.7	oz	Croutons	2.00	12.80	3.60	93.00
0.7	fl oz	Reduced-fat Italian salad dressing	0.04	0.00	0.00	6.26
2	each	Egg	13.40	2.60	14.60	200.00
1	large	Mixed garden salad	2.60	19.00	0.80	98.00
		Totals	**18.04**	**34.40**	**19.00**	**397.26**
PM Snack						
1	each	Nonfat yogurt	7.00	11.00	0.00	7.00
		Totals	**7.00**	**11.00**	**0.00**	**7.00**
Dinner						
2	oz	Ribeye steak, grilled, lean	18.84	0.00	3.60	108.27
0.5	cup	Brown rice	2.45	24.85	0.60	116.00
3	cup	Mixed vegetables	3.30	9.30	0.66	72.90
0.25	cup	Chunky salsa	1.00	4.05	0.10	17.48
		Totals	**25.59**	**38.20**	**4.96**	**314.65**
Evening Snack						
0.7	oz	Popcorn	2.56	0.90	0.00	68.80
		Totals	**2.56**	**0.90**	**0.00**	**68.80**
Actual Totals			**65.41**	**156.78**	**25.61**	**1203.31**
Actual Percentage of Total Calories			**23.35**	**56.05**	**20.60**	**100.00**

Table 2.4. 1200-Calorie, Gluten-Free Meal Plan, Example 2

QTY	Measure	Description	Protein (g)	Carbs (g)	Fats (g)	Calories
Breakfast						
0.25	cup	Avocado, pureed	1.15	4.25	8.80	92.50
2	slice	Gluten-free bread	4.20	21.40	6.60	174.00
1	cup	Strawberries	1.00	9.00	0.00	60.00
		Totals	**6.35**	**34.65**	**15.40**	**326.50**
AM Snack						
1	each	Banana, medium	1.20	26.70	0.60	105.00
		Totals	**1.20**	**26.70**	**0.60**	**105.00**
Lunch						
0.4	oz	Carrot, grated	0.64	8.24	0.13	35.00
3.5	oz	Chicken breast	23.00	0.00	1.60	110.00
1	each	Gluten-free corn tortillas	1.35	13.75	0.80	70.00
0.25	cup	Chunky salsa	1.00	4.05	0.10	17.48
1.4	oz	Spinach, raw	1.40	0.64	0.20	12.40
1	small	Tomato	1.00	5.70	0.40	26.00
Totals	**28.39**	**Totals**	**28.39**	**32.38**	**3.23**	**270.88**
PM Snack						
1	each	Apple	0.30	21.00	0.50	81.00
		Totals	**0.30**	**21.00**	**0.50**	**81.00**
Dinner						
0.25	cup	Brown rice, cooked	1.23	12.43	0.30	58.00
1	each	Tuna burger	30.28	14.75	4.36	221.13
2	cup	Mixed vegetables	2.20	6.20	0.44	48.60
4	tsp	Chunky salsa	0.00	6.00	0.00	20.00
		Totals	**33.71**	**39.38**	**5.10**	**347.73**
Evening Snack						
1	each	Nonfat yogurt	7.00	11.00	0.00	70.00
		Totals	**7.00**	**11.00**	**0.00**	**70.00**
Actual Totals			**76.95**	**165.11**	**24.84**	**1201.11**
Actual Percentage of Total Calories			**25.82**	**55.42**	**18.76**	**100.00**

Table 2.5. 1200-Calorie Vegetarian Meal Plan, Example 1

QTY	Measure	Description	Protein (g)	Carbs (g)	Fats (g)	Calories
Breakfast						
1	cup	Unsweetened almond milk	1.00	2.00	3.00	40.00
0.4	oz	Flax meal, flax seeds, or linseeds	3.60	0.80	1.20	33.00
1	cup	Frozen mango	0.70	17.50	0.00	75.00
1	scoop	100% whey protein isolate	26.00	0.30	0.30	109.00
		Totals	**31.30**	**20.60**	**4.50**	**257.00**
AM Snack						
2	each	Mandarin	1.00	11.00	0.20	56.00
		Totals	**1.00**	**11.00**	**0.20**	**56.00**
Lunch						
2	each	Egg (whole, incl. yolk)	13.40	2.60	14.60	200.00
1	large	Mixed garden salad	2.60	19.00	0.80	98.00
2.8	oz	Sweet potato, baked or steamed	1.60	16.56	0.00	72.00
		Totals	**17.60**	**38.16**	**15.40**	**370.00**
PM Snack						
1	each	Carrot, raw, medium	0.70	7.30	0.10	31.00
1.5	oz	Hummus, commercial	3.32	6.00	4.03	69.72
1	tsp	Low fat peanut butter	0.80	1.00	1.90	28.00
2	each	Wheat crackers	1.40	7.60	0.80	48.00
		Totals	**6.22**	**22.70**	**6.83**	**176.72**
Dinner						
1	each	Exotic vegetable soup*	4.47	8.95	0.93	116.08
3.5	oz	Tofu	13.20	0.00	8.03	139.34
		Total	**17.67**	**8.95**	**8.96**	**255.42**
Evening Snack						
1	each	Honey baked fruit berry supreme*	2.00	23.79	0.41	124.15
		Totals	**2.00**	**23.79**	**0.41**	**124.15**
Actual Totals			**75.79**	**125.20**	**36.30**	**1239.29**
Actual Percentage of Total Calories			**26.81**	**44.29**	**28.90**	**100.00**

Table 2.6. 1200-Calorie Vegetarian Meal Plan, Example 2

QTY	Measure	Description	Protein (g)	Carbs (g)	Fats (g)	Calories
Breakfast						
1.4	oz	Low-fat muesli	3.52	24.92	1.16	136.00
0.5	oz	Flax meal, flax seeds, or linseeds	5.40	1.20	1.80	49.50
1	cup	Strawberries	1.00	9.00	0.00	60.00
1	each	Nonfat yogurt	7.00	11.00	0.00	70.00
		Totals	**16.92**	**46.12**	**2.96**	**315.50**
AM Snack						
2	each	Mandarin	1.00	11.00	0.20	56.00
		Totals	**1.00**	**11.00**	**0.20**	**56.00**
Lunch						
0.7	fl oz	Reduced-fat Italian salad dressing	0.04	0.00	0.00	6.26
2	each	Egg	13.40	2.60	14.60	200.00
1	large	Mixed garden salad	2.60	19.00	0.80	98.00
		Totals	**16.04**	**21.60**	**15.40**	**304.26**
PM Snack						
1	each	Apple	0.30	21.00	0.50	81.00
1	scoop	100% whey protein isolate	26.00	0.30	0.30	109.00
0.5	cup	Water	0.00	0.00	0.00	0.00
		Total	**26.30**	**21.31**	**0.80**	**190.00**
Dinner						
1.5	each	Vegetable bake*	25.38	28.00	1.42	267.58
		Totals	**25.38**	**28.00**	**1.42**	**267.58**
Evening Snack						
0.7	oz	Popcorn, all natural	2.56	0.90	0.00	68.80
		Totals	**2.56**	**0.90**	**0.00**	**68.80**
Actual Totals			**88.20**	**128.93**	**20.78**	**1202.14**
Actual Percentage of Total Calories			**33.42**	**48.86**	**17.72**	**100.00**

Table 2.7. 1200-Calorie Vegan Meal Plan, Example 1

QTY	Measure	Description	Protein (g)	Carbs (g)	Fats (g)	Calories
Breakfast						
1	each	Banana, medium	1.20	26.70	0.60	105.00
0.4	oz	Flax meal, flax seeds, or linseeds	3.60	0.80	1.20	33.00
3.5	oz	Frozen mixed berries	1.20	9.30	0.00	47.00
0.9	oz	Pea protein	20.90	0.70	0.30	92.00
1	oz	Rolled oats	4.02	18.00	0.27	120.00
		Total	**30.92**	**55.50**	**2.37**	**397.00**
AM Snack						
2	each	Mandarin	1.00	11.00	0.20	56.00
		Totals	**1.00**	**11.00**	**0.20**	**56.00**
Lunch						
3.5	oz	Firm tofu	13.20	0.00	8.03	139.34
1	large	Mixed garden salad	2.60	19.00	0.80	98.00
3.5	oz	Sweet potato, baked or steamed	2.00	20.70	0.00	90.00
		Totals	**17.80**	**39.70**	**8.83**	**327.34**
PM Snack						
1	each	Carrot, raw, medium	0.70	7.30	0.10	31.00
1.5	oz	Hummus, commercial	3.32	6.00	4.03	69.72
		Totals	**4.02**	**13.30**	**4.13**	**100.72**
Dinner						
1	each	Exotic vegetable soup*	4.47	8.95	0.93	116.08
3.5	oz	Firm tofu	13.20	0.00	8.03	139.34
		Totals	**17.67**	**8.95**	**8.96**	**255.42**
Evening Snack						
1	each	Honey baked fruit berry supreme*	2.00	23.79	0.41	124.15
		Totals	**2.00**	**23.79**	**0.41**	**124.15**
Actual Totals			**73.41**	**152.24**	**33.74**	**1260.63**
Actual Percentage of Total Calories			**24.64**	**51.10**	**24.26**	**100.00**

Table 2.8. 1200-Calorie Vegan Meal Plan, Example 2

QTY	Measure	Description	Protein (g)	Carbs (g)	Fats (g)	Calories
Breakfast						
0.5	each	Banana, medium	0.60	13.35	0.30	52.50
0.4	oz	Flax meal, flax seeds, or linseeds	3.60	0.80	1.20	33.00
1	cup	Frozen mango	0.70	17.50	0.00	75.00
0.7	oz	Natural muesli	2.20	10.30	1.68	68.41
0.9	oz	Pea protein	20.90	0.70	0.30	92.00
		Totals	**28.00**	**42.65**	**3.48**	**320.91**
AM Snack						
2	each	Mandarin	1.00	11.00	0.20	56.00
		Totals	**1.00**	**11.00**	**0.20**	**56.00**
Lunch						
1	each	Super grain salad*	18.00	17.00	5.80	190.00
1	oz	Spinach, raw	1.05	0.48	0.15	9.30
		Totals	**19.05**	**17.48**	**5.95**	**199.30**
PM Snack						
1	each	Apple	0.30	21.00	0.50	81.00
0.9	oz	Pea protein	20.90	0.70	0.30	92.00
1	cup	Water	0.00	0.00	0.00	0.00
		Totals	**21.20**	**21.70**	**0.80**	**173.00**
Dinner						
1	each	Delicious vegetarian tofu*	21.20	38.90	11.20	356.20
		Totals	**21.20**	**38.90**	**11.20**	**356.20**
Evening Snack						
1	each	Honey baked fruit berry supreme*	2.00	23.79	0.41	124.15
		Totals	**2.00**	**23.79**	**0.41**	**124.15**
Actual Totals			**92.45**	**155.52**	**22.04**	**1229.56**
Actual Percentage of Total Calories			**31.32**	**52.68**	**16.00**	**100.00**

ACTION 12: MODIFYING YOUR DAILY MEAL PLAN

Based on the meal plans you have read through above, I'd like you to refer to the notes you made in action 11 and write down what surprised you about the meal plans. What concerns, if any, did you have reading through the meals?

_____

_____

_____

_____

_____

_____

_____

_____

Here are a few things I hear most often from clients when they first see their meal plans:

- Wow! Breakfast looks big.
- Six meals are a lot to eat. How can I lose fat if I'm eating more than I was before?
- That's a lot of vegetables.
- I can't fit six meals into my day. I don't get many breaks.
- It seems like so much food!

Trust me when I say I've heard it all before! Remember, you have invested in *Awaken the Sexy within* to make a change in your body, transforming it to a sexier version of yourself. The chances are, you cannot keep doing what you are currently doing and expect a different outcome. There simply must be changes. In every instance that I have worked with a client, even if they believe their food is on track, they need to change their way of eating to achieve the outcome they want. You will need to make changes too.

Consistency is the key. Measuring your portions in accordance with the meal plans is also essential for determining the volume of food you will be eating at each meal. Eating smaller, more frequent meals will keep your energy levels balanced throughout the day, ensure your blood sugar levels are maintained, and help you avoid cravings and binges.

ACTION 13: SELECTING YOUR NEW EATING LIFESTYLE

Using the above templates as a guide, I want you to select an option that is suitable for you based upon your fitness goals, your medical history (and appropriate consultation with your doctor), your you're your activity levels, and an approximation of your caloric intake. There are many calorie calculators available online to help you home in on the exact range for you, but here are some general guidelines based on gender and activity level.

Women
- Sedentary: 1000–1200 calories
- Moderately active: 1200–1500 calories
- Very active: 1400–1800 calories

Men
- Sedentary: 1200–1500 calories
- Moderately active: 1500–1800 calories
- Very active: 1800–2100 calories

Remember, the more active you are, the more calories you'll burn. It is always better to burn additional calories through exercise than to drastically reduce caloric intake by eating less. Please consult your doctor or physician before making any adjustments to your nutrition plan.

As a general guide, take the calories for your maintenance fat and subtract 500 calories to calculate your calories to achieve fat loss. Write down your calorie guidelines here.

My calculated number of calories per day to maintain my weight are

_____.

My calculated number of calories per day to achieve fat loss are

_____.

Make a note below as to the meal plans you have selected to use as guidelines for your new way of eating. Write down the adjustments that you will need to make, if any, to allow for the difference in calories. For instance, if you need to consume 1500 calories, that works out to be an additional 300 calories. My suggestion would be to look at the snacks and lunch or dinner meals and see how you can easily increase a couple by adding a piece of fruit, perhaps increasing some higher-energy food, such as the rice. Generally, you will only need to make a couple of adjustments. Doing so will help you really understand the numbers behind what you are eating and take more ownership over your outcomes.

Remember, I'm not asking you to count calories every day. Once you get your measurements accurately, you won't need to count. You will simply measure using approximations of weight and volume of foods, occasionally bringing in a kitchen scale to help. If you do not do this, you will find your serving sizes begin to creep out further and further.

Go ahead and write down the adjustments you'll make to your chosen meal plan here.

_____

_____

_____

_____

_____

_____

RECIPES

Chicken Stir Fry Supreme

Stir-frying is so quick and easy, and you can easily add lots of different colored vegetables to create amazing, flavorful meals. Another bonus is how well they freeze. A tip I always tell clients is to double up on all the ingredients and freeze the extra meals for later in the week.

Preparation Time: 15 minutes

Servings: 4

Ingredients

2 cups chicken breast fillets, diced

1 red onion, sliced

4 cups mixed vegetables, including broccoli, cauliflower, carrot, snap peas, Asian greens, red pepper

Juice of 1 lime

2 tbsp soy sauce,

3 tbsp hoisin, oyster, or black bean sauce

1 tbsp sweet chili sauce

1 tbsp honey

Method

Heat fry pan and spray with olive oil and heat. Place chicken and onion and cook over high heat until browned. Add all the remaining ingredients, apart from the vegetables, and cook for a further 2–5 min. Add all vegetables and cook for a further 5–7 minutes.

Nutritional Information

Per serving

Calories	271
Protein	35 g
Carbohydrates	11 g
Sugar	9.2 g

Fiber	12.5 g
Fat	5 g

Tuna Burgers

These tuna burgers are quick and easy to make, taste amazing, and freeze very well. They are great served with salad or fresh vegetables and a side of salsa.

Preparation Time: 15 minutes
Servings: 8 burgers

Ingredients

15 oz (1 can) tuna in water, drained

1 onion, finely chopped

1 tbsp fresh ginger, finely chopped

1 clove garlic, finely chopped

2 tbsp coriander, chopped

2 tbsp parsley or mint, chopped

Freshly ground black pepper

1 whole egg

¼ cup of whole wheat breadcrumbs

Canola oil spray

Method

Place all the ingredients in a bowl and mix well until they are all combined. Place a portion of the mixture into your palm and shape into a burger. My tip is to place them on a plate, cover with cling wrap, and leave in the fridge for at least 30 minutes to settle before cooking. I find that you get less breakage of the burgers if you follow this step first.

Heat fry pan and spray lightly with oil. Place burgers carefully into the pan as the burgers may crumble if you handle too roughly. Cook for approximately 3 minutes on each side.

Nutritional Information

Per serving (2 burgers)

Calories	158	Fiber	0.8 g
Protein	28 g	Fat	3 g
Carbohydrates	4 g	Saturated fat	0.8 g
Sugar	1.4 g		

Exotic Vegetable Soup

This soup is loaded with delicious vegetables and so incredibly quick and easy to make. Cost effective and very flexible. You will see a range of vegetables listed below, but feel free to substitute them with your favorites. Great for winter and storing extra servings in the freezer.

Preparation Time: 30 minutes

Servings: 8

Ingredients

500 g pumpkin, diced into cubes

4 stalks celery, sliced

4 cups broccoli or cauliflower

2 large carrots, sliced

1 large zucchini, diced

1 large red onion, chopped

2 garlic cloves, minced

8 cups reduced-salt vegetable stock

⅓ cup parsley, chopped

1 tsp curry powder

Black pepper to taste

Method

Combine all the ingredients into a large cooking pot once they've been washed and prepared. Bring the pot to the boil and simmer for 15–20 minutes.

Prior to serving, ensure the vegetables are cooked to your liking. If you prefer your soup blended, use a blending wand until all the ingredients are textured to your satisfaction. Otherwise, serve as a chunky soup, and enjoy!

Nutritional Information

Per Serving

Calories	153
Protein	5 g
Carbohydrates	29 g
Sugar	12 g

Fiber	5.3 g
Fat	1.1 g
Saturated fat	0.2 g

Honey Baked Fruit Berry Supreme

This is a delicious dessert that you can have for breakfast or snacks. It's so easy to make, takes no time, and freezes well for your convenience. I love to eat this one served with some low-fat, low-sugar yogurt.

Preparation Time: 35 minutes

Servings: 8

Ingredients

4 cups (about 2 lbs) apples, diced or sliced

18 oz frozen mixed berries

¼ cup of raisins

1 tbsp honey

Sprinkle ground cinnamon

1 cup natural muesli

Method

Preheat the oven to 350°F (180°C). Core and dice your apples and cut appropriately. You can use a combination of apples and pears if you prefer. Place the fruit into a baking dish, add the frozen mixed berries and raisins and mix until all ingredients are combined.

Drizzle honey across the top of the mixture, dust with cinnamon, and spread the natural muesli across the top of the dish. Cover with foil, and bake in the oven for 30 minutes.

Delicious served with the low-fat and low-sugar yogurt.

Nutritional Information

Per Serving

Calories	130		Fiber		5 g
Protein	1.7 g		Fat		1 g
Carbohydrates	27 g			Saturated fat	0.3 g
	Sugar	16.5 g			

Vegetable Bake

This is a family favorite. Using so many different varieties of vegetables, it's always a winner. Once again, it's great for the freezer, so make sure you make up a big batch. A tip I give people is to double the recipe, divide up the additional servings into separate containers, and freeze them for other days.

If you're looking for some condiments to have with it, try one of these: salsa, sweet chili sauce, or a low-fat, low-sugar chutney or relish.

Preparation Time: 20 minutes

Servings: 6

Ingredients

29 oz (2 cans) canned tomatoes

1 Spanish onion, finely sliced

1 cup frozen peas

2 cups mixed vegetables, such as broccoli, cauliflower, and carrot, chopped

2 cups fresh spinach

2 cups mushrooms, sliced

1 cup low-fat mozzarella cheese

1 cup brown rice, cooked

Method

Preheat the oven to 350°F (180°C). Spray a large baking tray with oil and then alternate layers of the spinach, rice, tomatoes, mixed vegetables, and cheese. Repeat this layering process until the baking dish is filled.

Cook for 15–20 minutes until the cheese is melted. This is delicious served hot or cold.

Nutritional Information

Per serving

Calories	190	Fiber		5.1 g
Protein	18 g	Fat		5.8 g
Carbohydrates	17 g		Saturated fat	3.3 g
Sugar	6.5 g			

Super Grain Salad

Don't you just love super grains? This great recipe, incorporating loads of mixed vegetables and herbs, is an incredibly delicious and nutritious meal.

Preparation Time: 20 minutes

Servings: 4

Ingredients

1 cup quinoa, uncooked

½ Spanish onion, chopped

2 cups carrots, diced

4 stalks celery, diced

1 red pepper, diced

1 handful chopped parsley

2 tbsp flaxseeds

2 tbsp chia seeds

Sauce

Juice of 1 lime

1 tbsp soy sauce

1 tsp sweet chili sauce

Method

Cook the quinoa and mix all the ingredients in it, allowing it to rest and cool. Mix together the sauce ingredients until they are combined. Pour over all combined ingredients when it's time to serve.

Nutritional Information

Per serving

Calories	215
Protein	8.2 g
Carbohydrates	41.2 g
Sugar	6.7 g

Fiber	5.3 g
Fat	3.3 g
Saturated fat	0.3 g

Delicious Vegetarian Tofu

This is one of the quickest and easiest salads to prepare. Amazing color with remarkable textures and a zesty flavor that will have you coming back for more.

Preparation Time: 7 minutes

Servings: 4

Ingredients

14 oz (1 package) tofu

2 cups mixed salad leaves

1 medium cucumber, diced

2 carrots, diced

2 celery sticks, sliced

½ cup corn kernels

¼ cup walnuts, diced

½ Spanish onion, diced

2 cups brown rice, cooked

2 tbsp red wine vinegar

1 tbsp Dijon mustard

Method

Combine all the ingredients, apart from the vinegar and mustard, into a large serving bowl and mix carefully until combined. In a separate bowl, combine the vinegar and mustard. You can experiment with different vinegars and mustards to find the dressing to suit your taste. Pour the dressing over the salad and mix to combine.

Nutritional Information

Per serving

Calories	356
Protein	21.2 g
Carbohydrates	38.9 g
Sugar	2 g

Fiber	14.2 g
Fat	11.2 g
Saturated fat	1 g

**DO NOT MOVE ON TO THE NEXT CHAPTER UNTIL YOU HAVE
COMPLETED EVERY ACTION ITEM ABOVE.
NO EXCUSES!**

Summary

- Consume six meals per day to help keep your metabolism elevated—breakfast, lunch, and dinner, along with a morning snack, afternoon snack, and evening snack.
- Timing your nutrition is crucial. Consume a meal every 2–3 hours once you've had your breakfast.
- A typical daily menu should contain the following, substituting vegetarian or vegan alternatives where required:

  Breakfast: Protein in the form of egg whites, a protein drink, or low-fat yogurt + some plant based food (e.g., fruits or vegetables) + some high-energy food (e.g., 1 cup of breakfast cereal or a piece of whole wheat toast).

  Morning Snack: A small tub of yogurt or a piece of fruit.

  Lunch: Protein in the form of chicken, salmon, or tuna (approximately 4 ounces) + a salad mix with lots of color and crunch. Or one round of sandwiches on whole wheat bread or one wrap with filled with 4 ounces of protein and salad.

  Afternoon Snack: Same as for morning snack.

  Dinner: Protein in the form of chicken, beef, fish, steak, or pork (approximately 4 ounces) + 3 cups of mixed colorful and crunchy vegetables + up to 1 cup of high-energy food such as cooked brown rice, pasta, or sweet potato.

  Evening Snack: Popcorn (½-ounce pack), a small piece of bread with some peanut butter or avocado, or a piece of fruit and some yogurt.

- Drink at least 50 fluid ounces of water (seven 8-ounce glasses) every day.
- Aim for 6 hours of sleep per night to help keep you energized.
- Commit to the new you and a healthy eating lifestyle!

SUCCESS STORY:
Kristy Whiting, 30 years old

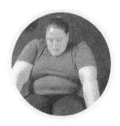
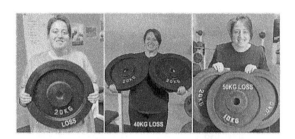

Kristy lost 110 pounds in 12 months, reducing her weight from 286 to 176 pounds. That's right: She lost an amazing 74 inches of fat from her waist, hips, chest, arms, and legs! An incredible achievement through focus and commitment to our never-fail nutrition and training approach to life-sustainable weight loss. Kristy has been driven to success by her hunger to win back her body. With only 33 pounds to go to reach her goal, we have been coaching Kristy to set some longer-term goals beyond her final weight loss target.

It's fair to say that Kristy is on fire and an amazing inspiration to everyone that has seen her transform.

"The mind, body, and soul transformational journey I've undergone with Robb has been an amazing experience, and I'm extremely grateful. Robb is a great coach and has designed a tailored nutritional plan along with an exercise training program that has made it possible to achieve my goals. Every step of the way, Robb has been there to help support, guide, motivate, and encourage me, consistently pushing me to prove to myself that I can and will exceed my expectations."

CHAPTER 3

Why Sexiness Must Be Tracked

To this point, you've got a plan, you've set goals, you have a set of meal plans to transform your eating, and you will shortly see the workouts that are going to help shape your body. But more is required to make your plan succeed completely. You need accountability! Accountability is *the* main reason that people use my services. With the right accountability comes results and transformation.

Accountability simply means accepting responsibility for our actions and acknowledging the results of those actions honestly. Let's break that down in the context of what it means for you in accomplishing your body transformation and optimizing your health. You must account for your activities. That means tracking what you do every step of the way. You must track what you eat, the physical activity you undertake, how much water you're drinking each day, how much sleep you're getting, and how you would rate your self-management in working toward your health and fitness goals. It sounds like a lot, but when you break it down into bite-size pieces, it's nowhere near as hard as it first may seem.

This is such a critical point to note. You will be seven to eight times more likely to succeed if you track each of the steps I've mentioned above. The clients of mine that do the best are almost religious about their tracking. It truly does work. Why? Because it keeps you so incredibly focused and on track. When you know you must write things down, it keeps you concentrated on what you should be doing. For instance, when you follow one of the meal plans, you know you need to measure the servings to be accurate, and knowing that you need to write it down makes you more likely to adhere to it. Sometimes, we avoid exercises like this because we know we'll feel guilty if we stray from the plan. But you made a plan because you want to see transformation. If you don't do your best to follow it by tracking your progress, you'll be letting yourself down.

The trouble is that, as humans, we don't like to fail. We don't like to feel pain. We go easy on ourselves and find ways to justify mediocrity to ourselves. For instance, "I was close enough to achieving what I wanted. I'm pretty much sticking to the entire plan." The harsh truth is you either do it or you don't. There's no in between.

You need to use that pain to drive you to work harder to achieve what you want. Remember it's what *you* want. Why wouldn't you achieve it? Because you don't want it bad enough? You think it will take too much hard work? You haven't been able to do it before, so why will now be any different? You like food too much? You feel you'll have to give up too much?

Do some of those excuses sound familiar?

Our Greatest Strengths Can Also Be Our Greatest Weaknesses

We have been programmed with a special feature. It is one of our greatest strengths but also one our greatest weaknesses. It's our ability to remove ourselves from pain. This is a crucial feature of our nervous system and allows us to, for instance, quickly remove our hand from a hot surface we touch by accident. We have been provided this gift by our creator so that we don't physically injure ourselves.

However, pain can also work against us, even though working through that pain would benefit us in the long term. For example, we remove ourselves from painful situations that involve our emotions. We feel pain because we believe something will be too difficult or painful to face that emotion or work through it. For example, a work colleague who you find disruptive and distracting needs to understand the impact that they are having on your work. However, you don't want to talk to them because you worry your conversation could lead to confrontation, which would be stressful and painful for you. So, instead, you choose to say nothing and maybe even find a new job over time.

Another example could relate more closely to your health and fitness. You have 45 pounds (20 kilograms) to lose and know how amazing you will feel when you reach your goal. You'll have increased energy, and your clothes will feel better on you. But, instead, you think about all the times you've failed before, all the questions you have about how to achieve results, how much you'll miss the foods you love to eat, and the sore muscles in your future. I'm sure you can think of a similar example in your own mind.

We just don't naturally like pain, whether it's physical or emotional!

However, we humans have another amazing gift, which is the ability to push through pain to achieve a greater outcome. I like to call this increasing our "emotional fitness." In the examples I've listed above, the problems would have been resolved if the individuals pushed against the resistance they were feeling and just did the work required.

What happens each time you do a push-up? The first time you do it, you might struggle. The next time will be a little better. The more times you do a push-up, the better equipped you are physically to keep doing them. Your body is physiologically adapting and responding to the resistance you are placing upon it. You can't just do one push-up and expect your chest muscles to grow in a way that enables you to do 100 push-ups whenever you like. You must put the muscles under a huge amount of resistance to stimulate that amount of muscle growth.

Well guess what? Your emotional fitness is the same. When you are in positions of emotional discomfort, there is an opportunity to do one of two things. The first is to do nothing. The second is to push against the resistance and pain you are feeling to get to the other side. When you first do this, it will be very hard, just like the push-up. But as you push against more and more emotional resistance, you are building more and more emotional muscle. Over time, you become emotionally fitter. It isn't about the outcome you achieve, but it is about who you become along the way to your outcome that truly matters.

Think of the most painful times in your life and how they have helped you grow. If I think of the times when I was bullied, I can recall the years of pain and anguish I suffered as a result. But when I made the decision to change my body and mindset, I pushed against the emotional pain to help myself achieve the incredible life I lead today. It is not about who I am now. It is who I became during this journey from surviving to thriving that changed my world.

ACTION 14: IDENTIFYING YOUR PAIN, FEAR, AND DOUBT

I want to check in with where you are right now. Think of a recent time when you were faced with something that was emotionally painful and challenging for you. Write it down.

_____

_____

_____

_____

_____

Write down the emotions you felt and the actions you took or wish you'd taken to overcome them.

_____

_____

_____

_____

_____

_____

_____

Write down what the outcomes of those actions and inactions.

_____

_____

_____

_____

_____

_____

Did you have the outcome you wanted? Write down what else you could have done to improve the outcome.

_____

_____

_____

_____

_____

_____

_____

_____

_____

_____

_____

_____

Change requires courage. If you're reading this now, my presumption is that you want to change. That's an incredible start. You've decided you need to change. The next steps—which most people don't take—are to commit to the decision, no matter what, then act until the change has occurred. It sounds so simple, yet most people simply don't do it.

You know the outcome of doing nothing. No change, except manifesting itself a little worse with the passing of each day as you create stories for yourself about what it all means for you. Be brave. Take a leap of faith. Be your own hero, and face your fears, your demons and greatest challenges. You will not regret the journey. There's a stronger, more focused and committed version of you on the other side.

Acknowledging Your Past Failures

Challenges, setbacks, and failures are such powerful gifts to us. Everything happens for a reason, and there are growth and learning opportunities in any situation where we feel we've failed. Sometimes, they can seem hard to find, but if you look, there is growth and goodness. The key is being focused to look and find it rather than ignore it and complain about it.

Focusing on your health and fitness, I want to spend some time considering your past—specifically, your past failures in health and fitness. I have had them before, so I am sure you have as well. We are going to walk through a process that identifies and acknowledges the failures and will use those failures as fuel for your success to come. You may not necessarily see how this links together right now, but you will by the time we get to the end. Have faith!

ACTION 15: IDENTIFYING THE REASONS YOU'VE FAILED IN THE PAST

Why did you fail with your health and fitness? Write down all the reasons you have failed.

_____

_____

_____

_____

_____

_____

_____

_____

What are some excuses you've come up with in the past to justify why you haven't succeeded?

_____

_____

_____

_____

_____

_____

Becoming Your Own Hero

Great job! Remember, your past does not represent your future, unless you decide to live there. This is your time. No more excuses. You must do things differently this time. Why? The definition of insanity is doing the same things over and over, expecting a different result. Assuming you're not insane and that you want a different outcome, let's begin identifying what those changes need to be. They may be big changes or slight adjustments; I don't know, but you will.

Before you complete the next action item embracing change, consider the examples below to prompt your thinking:

- Establishing a schedule of when to exercise
- Following a tailored meal plan
- Completing enough resistance training and cardio
- Tracking what you're doing for exercise and food
- Drinking enough water—more than 50 fluid ounces (7 glasses)
- Getting enough sleep
- Taking time to do your meal preparation.

- Sticking to your schedule
- Clearly articulating your goals, displaying them, referring to them on a regular basis

ACTION 16: EMBRACING CHANGE

List at least 10 things you *must* do differently this time for your health and fitness to avoid your past failures and ensure 100% success.

_____

_____

_____

_____

_____

_____

_____

11 Reasons Tracking What You Do Is Fundamental to Success

There's a high probability that if you feel you've failed in the past, you haven't tracked what it is you were doing on a day-to-day basis with your food and exercise. Tracking what you do each day is fundamental to your success for 11 reasons:

1. You will be more engaged in the action you take daily.

2. It creates focus and energy.

3. You will be more engaged with the lifestyle choices you make.

4. You can see what you're doing each day and the progress you're making will help motivate you.

5. You're making yourself accountable. The act of writing down your choices with food and exercise will make you more likely to comply with your plan.

6. If you have a coach who reviews your nutrition journal on a daily or weekly basis, it creates a high level of compliance. You will not want to write down your poorer food choices, so you're less likely to consume them. This is more powerfully true if you've agreed with your coach on consequences for noncompliance with your meal plan.

7. We don't like to fail. The act of being honest with yourself and accurate in the documentation of your behaviors, engages a level of discipline. It's painful to write down that you may have failed, so we tend to be compliant instead.

8. We often don't realize how far we've come until we look back. The process of looking back gives you an opportunity to celebrate your success and examine the challenges. Motivation, drive, focus, and inspiration are created through this process. When you track what you've been doing, it is easier to undertake this reflection.

9. It will help you reenergize and reengineer your focus on your goals.

10. Testing and measuring your results and what you have been doing creates power and direction.

11. You will be seven to eight times more likely to succeed if you track what you eat and drink, your exercise, the number of hours you sleep, and a rating of your management of your own health and fitness plan.

ACCOUNTABILITY TOOLS

Tool 1: The Empowerability Checklist

What's powerful about this tool is that it's a one-page dashboard inventory of your daily and weekly health and fitness. At a glance, you can see how well you're doing each day. It's simple and efficient and gives you all you need to track your progress. I've provided a copy of the checklist below with the first line completed as an example.

You'll need to print these checklists out, one copy for each week. Go to AwakenTheSexyWithin.com to print additional copies. You must keep them on display where you can see them multiple times per day to complete, and you must complete each section. Most sections require only a check mark if you've completed it. Either you have done what is required or you haven't. It's that black and white. Complete all sections of the form. No excuses!

WEEKLY EMPOWERABILITY CHECKLIST

Week beginning _____

Day	1. Eaten Nutritious Meals and Completed Your Daily Nutrition Log?						2. Vitamin Supplements	3. Water Intake (50+ fl oz)	4. Resistance Training	5. Cardio (20–45 min)	6. 10,000+ Steps	7. Rehab or Stretch Exercises	8. Sleep 6+ hours	9. Rate Your Plan Mgt (1–10)
	1	2	3	4	5	6								
Mon	√	√	√	√	√	√	√	1.8	–	Bike 20min	11.2k	√	5.5 hours	9.5
Tues														
Wed														
Thurs														
Fri														
Sat														
Sun														

ACTION 17: ACT NOW

Go to AwakenTheSexyWithin.com, and print out multiple copies of the checklist to start using immediately.

Tool 2: Nutrition Journal

Your nutrition journal is used to provide a more detailed breakdown of what you eat each day—every single food, every single quantity, every measure. It is critical that you complete this accurately. That means weighing your foods and using measuring cups to get the amounts just right. Take a few additional moments with each meal to ensure you get these fundamental components correct.

You must be able to take control of your results. You must take ownership of the details. If you don't, you won't be able to look back on what you have been doing and determine what to tweak or do completely differently.

My research shows that, generally, we will underestimate the quantity of food we eat by 10%–20% and will overstate the amount and intensity of exercise by up to 25%. Just remember, you're only cheating yourself if you don't accurately record your actions. Accuracy is crucial. Get it right the first time!

Below is a sample copy of the nutrition journal. Here is your link to download further copies: AwakenTheSexyWithin.com. Just like your empowerability checklist, you must keep them on display where you can see them multiple times per day to complete, and you must complete each section with full details of the meals you have eaten.

Although I don't ask any of my clients to count calories, I do ask you to be calorie aware. That means writing down the calories for your protein, carbs, and fats so that you can start to educate yourself about what you are eating. Write down the calories of some poorer food choices, and you'll quickly see how they compare to healthy and nutritious foods. When you gain an understanding of how hard you need to work to burn a certain number of calories, you will start to make different choices.

To provide you with an illustration as to how important it is to track what you're eating, I want you to refer to the table below to understand what is required in work effort to burn off the calories consumed. Once you grasp the concepts of energy in and energy out, you will realize the value of consistently maintaining an accurate record of your food in your nutrition journal. As you will see, it takes more time than you would think to burn off those unwanted calories. Awareness of this can make you more accountable to what you eat.

Food	Calories (Energy In)	Exercise	Minutes Required (Energy Out)
Blueberry muffin, large	589	Walking Jogging Cycling	164 68 90
Spaghetti Bolognese, 14 oz	526	Walking Jogging Cycling	146 60 80
McDonald's Big Mac	521	Walking Jogging Cycling	145 60 80
Sweet and sour chicken, 12 oz	459	Walking Jogging Cycling	128 53 70
McDonald's large fries	366	Walking Jogging Cycling	102 42 56
McDonald's hot fudge sundae, small	349	Walking Jogging Cycling	97 40 53
Fried rice, 1 cup	336	Walking Jogging Cycling	94 39 51
Hawaiian pizza, 2 slices	313	Walking Jogging Cycling	87 36 48
McDonald's large Coke	283	Walking Jogging Cycling	79 32 43
Krispy Kreme glazed doughnut	255	Walking Jogging Cycling	71 29 39
Hershey's Cookies 'n' Crème, 1.5 oz	220	Walking Jogging Cycling	61 25 34
Spring rolls, 3 oz	200	Walking Jogging Cycling	56 23 31
Beer, 13 oz	140	Walking Jogging Cycling	39 16 21
Chocolate chip cookie	81	Walking Jogging Cycling	22 12 9

Daily Nutrition Journal

Studioz

Date: _____

Personal Training

Description	Protein (grams)	Protein (calories)	Carbs (grams)	Carbs (calories)	Fats (grams)	Fats (calories)	Total Calories
Meal 1 (breakfast)							
Totals							
Meal 2 (am snack)							
Totals							
Meal 3 (lunch)							
Totals							
Meal 4 (pm snack)							
Totals							
Meal 5 (dinner)							
Totals							
Meal 6 (evening snack)							
Totals							
Daily Totals							
Goal Total							
Difference							

How much water did you drink today?   Was it enough?

Did you take your vitamins & supplements today?

How would you rate yourself onn management to your plan today (scale of 1 to 10, with 10 being the best)?

ACTION 18: ACT NOW

Go to AwakenTheSexyWithin.com, and print out multiple copies of the nutrition journal to start using immediately.

Tool 3. My Nutrition Coach App

The My Nutrition Coach app is available to you if you have one of our individually tailored meal plans. You require a sign on and password to access its functionality. It's a separate investment but truly worth it.

The app is very fast for tracking your food and can be completed with a few simple clicks. What is also great about the app is that you can sync it with the cloud with a click of a button, and our team can review it and discuss necessary changes with you during a coaching and accountability session.

Which version is best—manual or electronic app? Honestly, it is simply a matter of personal preference. Some people like the paper version, because they can see it, touch it, feel it. Others prefer the app, because it's convenient, you can update it anywhere, and it saves time in completing it. Personally, I use both. There are times when I love to keep the tracking in the app, so it's with me all the time. Other times, I print out the journal and have it on the side of my desk, so it's right under my nose all day long.

Both are equally powerful. You must have a hunger, focus, and drive to keep tracking. You know it will take you closer to your goals, much faster.

ACTION 19: ACT NOW

If you don't like the manual version of the nutrition journal, and you've got one of our individually tailored meal plans, you can use our app, My Nutrition Coach, available in both iTunes and Google Play stores. If you'd like us to prepare an individually tailored meal plan you can contact us via www.StudiozPT.com.au.

Tool 4: Coaching Is Your Fastest Route to Success

The highest-performing people in the world have coaches. It doesn't matter whether it's an athlete or a businessperson, the people who perform at the highest level will have multiple coaches to keep them accountable and to keep them driving forward.

A coach will help you get the result you want, faster. Your coach will hold you accountable to achieving your goals. Your coach will help establish your goals with you. Your coach will identify an individually tailored, workable plan for you. Your coach will be completely focused on what you need to move you closer to the results you want. Your coach will be available to answer any questions you have and help overcome obstacles in your way. Your coach will have a track record of delivering results that you want. Your coach will become a key member of your success team and will always have your back. You can redeem your FREE 45-minute coaching session by registering at www.StudiozPT.com.au.

ACTION 20: ACT NOW—FIND YOUR COACH

Write a list of at least three people that you would like to have as your personal coach. Write down the reasons that you have selected them, and circle your preferred coach once you've investigated their services and suitability to supporting you in achieving your health and fitness goals. Contact the coach and organize how to get started. If they are not located nearby or you cannot afford their services, follow them on social media, sign up for their newsletter, or look for other ways to interact with them. Remember, we can coach you from anywhere in the world if you're looking for a world-class coach with a proven track record of delivering life-changing results. You can get started with your free sexy bonuses, available with *Awaken the Sexy within.*

_____

_____

_____

_____

_____

ACTION 21: ACT NOW—GET ACCESS TO ROBBEVANS365.COM

Daily coaching via podcast is an effective approach to mind-feeding you to set your day up for success. I suggest you listen to motivating, inspiring, and educational content each morning. You can access my podcast series at www.RobbEvans365.com or across all the popular streaming platforms, including iTunes and Spotify. It's completely FREE and available now!

Tool 5: Letters to Accountability Partners
This tool is so powerful that it is not for the fainthearted. This is for you, the person 100% committed to seeing change. I want you to select three to five people in

your life that you can 100% absolutely count on, to keep you accountable to your new healthy, sexy habits you are embedding into your daily life.

I'm talking about someone you can count on to check in with you to see how you are doing. To push you to keep on going when it seems tough. To push you outside your comfort zone. To support you in your new healthy food choices. To encourage you to find a better version of yourself.

Often, that can mean stepping outside your current circle of family and friends to find those people. I have this saying: If you want to know who your friends are, try losing weight. Not everyone is as supportive as you'd like to think. Select people that will be rock solid in their support of you and your goals. Choose wisely!

Once you have selected your team, it's time to send them a letter asking them to support you. I prefer a letter over email or social media, because it shows that you've gone to more effort. You've committed yourself to paper, you've printed it, put it in an envelope, and posted it. It will make a very pleasant surprise for them in the mailbox when most of the mail they usually receive will be junk mail and bills!

Please read the sample accountability letter below in detail before I explain why it is incredibly powerful.

Dear Jane,

The reason that I am writing to you is that I'm on a mission to reach an amazing fitness and weight loss goal, and I want you to help keep me accountable. I have so much respect for you, and I know you can be my rock in keeping me on track. I want you to be a key member of my team.

When a person is accountable to someone else for doing what they said they would do, they act. After years of making excuses, they reach their goals and find what they've always wanted. I am ready to make the changes I need to be successful in my health and fitness journey.

The power of social expectation is very strong. If I tell others that I am going to do something, I make sure that I do it. But this is more than just talk; I know that I must take specific actions to achieve my goals. Here are my health and fitness goals that I am committing to:

[The following are examples. Please insert your specific commitments. You must be able to quantify your goals and place a completion date next to them.]

1. I will lose 30 pounds of fat by 25 December 2021.
2. I will improve my fitness assessment test results, as documented in *Awaken the Sexy within*, by at least 50% by 25 December 2021.

I am specifically committing to the following actions to achieve my health and fitness goals:

[Insert your specific commitments, but I have provided some examples.]

1. Three resistance workouts per week from *Awaken the Sexy within*
2. Four cardio workouts per week of at least 20 min each
3. Eat six healthy and nutritious meals per day following my meal plan
4. Complete my nutrition journal daily
5. Drink at least 50 ounces of fresh water each day
6. Sleep for at least 6 hours each day

This is where you come in, Jane. I would like you to check up on me from time to time to see how I am tracking toward my fitness goals. Trust me when I say this is going to create an incredible amount of focus from me!

So here is what I would like you to do:

1. Contact me within 24 hours of receiving this letter and discuss the specific actions that I've outlined above.
2. Discuss how and when you will help keep me accountable.
3. Discuss and agree with me the consequences of not achieving my daily actions.

4.   Discuss whether there is anything that you'd like me to hold you accountable to. We can be accountability buddies!

Every 4 weeks, I am going to send you an update as to my progress. Focus is critical for me, Jane, so please help me stay on track and accountable to myself and to you. Achieving my health and fitness goals is very important to me.

I look forward to hearing from you very soon, Jane.

Yours sincerely,

ROBB EVANS
Ph: 0421 123 456

You can download a copy of this letter to edit for your accountability partners at AwakenTheSexyWithin.com.

This is such a powerful tool. It requires you to step way outside your comfort zone and tell someone else what it is you want to achieve for your health and fitness and then ask them to hold you accountable. It is probably not too hard to see why most people will not want to do this step, is it?

Most people will never discuss with anyone else what it is they truly want for their health and fitness. They fear the possibility of failure. Then, if they don't achieve their goals, they don't have to have an awkward discussion with someone about why they have failed. We humans have a funny way of justifying mediocrity to ourselves so that we don't live in a state of emotional pain.

When I've discussed this strategy with people in the past, it surprises me when they say, "I'm not doing that." I remind them that they just told me how desperate they were to lose weight and change their life. "Why wouldn't you want to do it?" I ask. Those who resist this exercise tend to stay the same. In their minds, they've made the decision not to commit fully to change, which is why they don't want to share their goals with anyone. They don't want anyone else to know that they've failed.

Take a stand for yourself. Commit to your health and fitness goals. Commit to your accountability partner. This is another tool in your kit to make you 100% guaranteed of success. You do not have as much to lose as it feels. Just go for it!

ACTION 22: ACT NOW—IDENTIFYING YOUR SUPPORT TEAM

Write a list of three to five people who you will send letters. Now download the letters at AwakenTheSexyWithin.com, then edit, print, sign, and send the letters today!

_____

_____

_____

_____

_____

Tool 6: Working Out with a Buddy

Working out with others is a great way to stay motivated and keep your energy high for the duration of the workout. Most clients that train in our boot camps tell me that there's no way they would have pushed themselves this hard if they had simply done the workout by themselves. Some people have a naturally competitive nature; others like to coach and motivate during a session so that each person pushes to a higher level. Often, if you're feeling a little flat and lethargic, the other people around you can raise your intensity levels.

Beyond the workouts, you can engage each other in discussion about your meal plans and the obstacles you're facing. It's a great initiative to involve close friends, family, your partner, or your kids if they are completely supportive. In the incredibly busy lifestyles we lead, working out with your partner is a great way to stay connected away from the hustle and bustle of our day.

ACTION 23: ACT NOW—FIND YOUR BUDDY

Brainstorm a list of people that you would like to have as your workout buddy. Write down the reasons that you have selected them, and circle your preferred three buddies to support you in achieving your health and fitness goals. Contact each buddy, and organize how to get started.

_____

_____

_____

_____

Tool 7: Social Media Accountability

Similar to writing letters to accountability partners, you can make a commitment on social media to your community about your health and fitness goals. You can post video diaries, photos, commentary about your successes and challenges. You can post daily or weekly to track your progress and allow others to comment and encourage you.

Social media can invite comparisons and guilt for not achieving the same results as others. However, finding the right online fitness community for you can have powerful effects. Facebook has countless fitness groups you could join. Check to see if there are any in your area that focus on the workouts you enjoy. Instagram is another option. You can create a fitness-specific account and share progress photos. Using fitness-related hashtags can bring in a community of support and encouragement, and you can use those same hashtags to pay it forward and support others.

There's no reason to post things online to people who will not be supportive of your fitness journey. So if you don't think your current community will support you, build a new one.

Used effectively, this is another powerful tool to ensure your success.

ACTION 24: ACT NOW—SELECTING YOUR SOCIAL MEDIA PLATFORM

Write a list of the social media platforms that you would like to use as an accountability tool. Find a social media group where you feel safe and supported. You can find our Facebook page, Studioz Personal Training and Pakenham Boot Camps for Women. Start posting; we'd love to hear from you!

———————————————————————

———————————————————————

———————————————————————

———————————————————————

———————————————————————

Tool 8: Keeping a journal

I believe in writing down all that you want to achieve in your life. Already in *Awaken the Sexy within*, I've asked you to stop and write down what you want for your health and fitness, why it is important to you, how committed you are, what you've eaten in the last 24 hours, and a range of other things.

Why have I asked you to do those things?

A journal of your thoughts is very powerful, allowing you to track your own personal journey. It's not something that you need to share with anyone else; it can be private for you. It could be a short video each day or week, talking about where you are succeeding, what results you are achieving, and how you can keep moving forward through the challenges. It is not until we stop and look back that we realize how far we have come. When you can go back and read or watch what you wrote on day 1 and compare that to today, you'll see how far you have come in your journey. This can be motivating and can even give you a kick up the backside when you need it. Remember, consistency is the key. I suggest daily works best, even if you only record a few sentences.

ACTION 25: ACT NOW—STARTING YOUR JOURNAL

Select which approach you will take to record your journal—written or video. If you don't already have a notebook or a camera ready, start writing here.

_____

_____

_____

_____

A Final Point on Accountability

One of our biggest reasons for failure is not acting—not following through on the goals we set for ourselves. If that has been you in the past, we need to help you change that. Use each of these accountability tools to set yourself up for success. If you are naturally fearful of change, you need to remember that if you always do what you have always done, you will keep getting the results you have always gotten.

If you want a different result, you need to change what you've been doing. These tools will support you in your journey. They will make you feel uncomfortable from time to time, but that is what you need. If you are comfortable all the time, you will not grow. If you do not grow, you will not succeed.

I believe in you. Believe in yourself. Go forth, keep yourself accountable, and conquer!

DO NOT MOVE ON TO THE NEXT CHAPTER UNTIL YOU HAVE COMPLETED EVERY ACTION ITEM ABOVE. NO EXCUSES!

Summary

- Accountability is a critical key to your success.
- You must identify the pain of past health and fitness failures.
- You must embrace change and become your own hero.
- You must understand the power of the 11 reasons that tracking what you do each day is fundamental to your success.
- Use the eight powerful accountability tools to enable you to reach your health and fitness goals sooner with guaranteed success.

SUCCESS STORY:
Ron Smelter, 54 years old

Ron lost 51 pounds (a 22% weight loss), reduced his body fat by 12.9%, and lost a total of 32 inches from his chest, waist, hips, arms, and thighs.

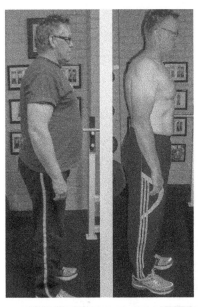

"I thought I needed to do something about my health and fitness when I was on a business trip overseas and saw a photo of myself sitting in a chair. I was also feeling very uncomfortable in my clothes, and I kept going up in sizes as my weight kept climbing. High blood pressure was also a problem for me, and I also lacked energy. I was feeling fat, had no energy at the end of the day, and could not be bothered doing anything once I was home from work.

"When I think about the results I've achieved, I feel great. Getting the weight off and getting my body back in shape has been great, but best of all, my health is good, my blood pressure is down to safe levels, I have heaps of energy, and I don't like sitting around anymore. I feel like I need to do something and get out and enjoy life. I've enjoyed getting back into bike riding. Now, I love the training. It's just part of my life.

"Training with Robb has helped change my life. I feel that I now have the tools and knowledge to carry me through life. I feel like I've now struck the right balance between my working life and health. I've put myself first, so that I can make sure my health doesn't spiral out of control, while still getting my work done.

"One other great thing has come out of my training: My wife has seen the results, she is very happy, and she tells me I am hot—which feels great! She has now started training with Robb and has also achieved amazing results. Thanks for everything, Robb."

CHAPTER 4

How to Overcome All Obstacles

Some of you may be at the beginning of your transformation journey, while others may be well on their way. Success in your sexiness journey requires focus and a hunger for a new version of you. No matter where you are in the journey, we all have thing in common: Our individual journeys will not be the same. You're all different, your goals will be different, and your lives are different. But you all crave a sexier version of yourself. That hunger you have is an amazing gift. Don't lose it. Be grateful for it. One thing I can tell you for sure is that, as soon as you lose that hunger and drive, progress and results will suffer.

Hunger creates focus, drive, motivation, and energy to move any obstacle that lays in your way. It's so easy to come up with excuses for why things are the way they are, why you can't have the body you want, and determining all the reasons it is just too hard for *you*.

Let's do an exercise right now.

ACTION 26: EMPOWERING YOUR SEXINESS

Create a list of all the reasons and excuses you can identify that may prevent you from having the amazing, sexy body you deserve. Be honest! You don't have to share this with anyone; it's an inner conversation with you and yourself. For example, not enough time, too tired, too lazy, unmotivated, unsupportive spouse, too expensive, too dark outside, too cold, too hot, don't have the equipment. Your turn.

_____

_____

_____

_____

_____

_____

_____

_____

Limits Imposed by Yourself

The only way to move forward is to bust through the limiting beliefs you have. There's a saying that I first heard from Tony Robbins: "Your past does not represent your future." I love this because so many of us continue to live in the past and use the outcomes of those past events to dictate what our future holds, holding you back from progress in all aspects of your life. Your past will only determine your future if you allow it to and choose to live there. It is time for you to have courage, to stand up for yourself like you never have before. Make today the new beginning of your empowered sexiness journey to your ultimate mind and body.

One of my limiting beliefs when I was a teenager and young adult, was that I was too short and too ugly for any girl to fall in love with me and want to share time with me. You see, during high school, a large portion of the kids around me had girlfriends, and I didn't. There were girls I wanted to date, but the ones I asked said they weren't interested. As more rejections came, the more withdrawn I became. My confidence sank, and my fears and insecurities grew. Every time I thought of asking someone out, I told myself, "Why bother? Everyone has said no before. Why would this time be different?"

I lived this way for over 10 years and didn't have my first girlfriend until I was 23 years old. I felt like I had missed out on an important milestone of adolescence. Could I have found a wonderful girl to date before I was in my 20s? Maybe, but I was too afraid to ask. I let my limiting beliefs keep me down for much too long.

It's crucial that you believe change and focus are achievable. Trust me. Limiting beliefs, frankly, suck. Several years ago, I made an important decision. It was to raise the standards in every area of my life to create a better version of myself for myself, my children, my clients, my family, and all the people whose lives I touch. I focused and acted to make progress every single day. No exceptions.

It's now time once again for you to act. Keeping in mind the task you completed in action 26, I want you to create a list of ways in which you can completely crush and eliminate each limiting belief from your life. For each limiting belief, I want you to create at least five ways you can eliminate it. Don't think that I underestimate how challenging this task will be for you. It may take you a few hours or even days to do it justice. But do not move forward in the book without doing this. It will limit your success if you don't. This is where you need to be strong and have faith in the process. If you spend the time and do it properly, you will create an unstoppable version of yourself.

To give an example of this exercise, my limiting belief was, "I will never be in a loving relationship because I'm too short and too ugly, and I have nothing to offer."

How I eliminated the limiting beliefs was to identify emotional and empowering phrases that reshaped my mindset into what I wanted to achieve. Not just one, but 11 powerful statements that resonated with my entire physiology, heart, and mind:

1. If you treat others as you want to be treated, people will love and respect you.

2. You are an incredibly loving and amazing soul; you will attract women by letting them see the real you.

3. Do what you love with all the passion and energy you have, and you will find the right person who wants to share that journey with you.

4. Always show up with the love, energy, fun, and playfulness that you want in your partner, and you will attract that person into your life.

5. Believe in yourself, because you can do anything you set your mind to.

6. The past does not represent your future. You will create the absolute best version of yourself with passion. You will focus every day to make yourself better today than yesterday.

7. There are many things in your life that you cannot control. But you can always be in control of what things mean to you.

8. All things happen for a reason. If you're not in a relationship, there is more growth for you required before your soul mate comes to you.

9. You cannot control the love you receive, but you are in complete control of the love you give. You feel loved by giving love. If you give more love to others, you will feel more loved. You are therefore in complete control of how much love you want to feel.

10. Relax, do what you love, be yourself, love yourself, be true to your heart and soul. Your destiny awaits.

11. When people discover your inner beauty, it will not matter at all what you look like on the outside. Your height, your perceptions of your facial features and body have no meaning when people see your inner gifts.

In your next action item below, I've asked you to identify five reasons your limiting belief isn't true. If I can come up with eleven, you can certainly come up with at least five. The more you write, the more likely you are to crush those limiting beliefs and create powerful, empowering, passionate, and meaningful statements. The 11 I created had a dramatic impact on my mindset. Rather than telling myself that I wasn't worthy of a relationship, I came up with statements that essentially said the complete opposite. I didn't change the physical me. I just knew that I definitely couldn't attract love if I couldn't feel it for myself. After all, if I didn't see those qualities, how could I expect anyone else to?

Go forth and conquer this task until you believe in yourself and that your created statements inspire you to create a new version of yourself.

ACTION 27: CRUSHING YOUR LIMITING BELIEFS

Okay, no more hesitation, I'm sure you have a strong mindset about what is required for this task. It's your turn. Write down at least five ways you can crush each limiting belief you identified in action 26. Make sure you use powerful and emotive language that inspires you to break through and be free of this baggage of the past. Life is too short to settle.

_____

_____

_____

_____

_____

_____

_____

Limits Imposed by Others

We have talked about the limiting beliefs you place on yourself, but what about the limits placed on you by others? I want you to think about the following people in your life:

- Your partner (if you are currently in a relationship, if not think about your previous relationship)
- Your children (if applicable)

- Your parents
- Your grandparents
- Your extended family
- Your friends
- Your social media friends or followers on Facebook, Twitter, Instagram, Snapchat, LinkedIn, YouTube, etc.
- Your work colleagues
- Your neighbors
- People you run into regularly (e.g., the person who always runs the register at the grocery store)
- Any person that you encounter from time to time

Considering all those people and all the interactions you have with them, do you feel that any of them talk to you in a way that denigrates how you feel about yourself? My work with thousands of clients shows me that almost everyone has someone who does this. Usually, when I ask, I get a response like, "Hell yeah! There's someone on Facebook who makes me feel terrible." Often, it's a partner, parent, or relative that makes a comment that can cut deep.

Body transformation is an emotional process. People are always willing to give you their advice about which diet you should follow or how what you are doing isn't right. Yet, the reality is, the person telling you has no training or experience in body transformation. Oftentimes, they are struggling through their own transformation.

So why do they do it? What do you think they're doing when they're saying these things to you?

People love to impose their limiting beliefs on to you because they don't want you to change. And they don't want you to change because it may make them feel bad about themselves or because they don't want to be asked to keep up. They want to stay where they are. But you don't. Put simply, some people would rather see you fail than succeed. In that way, they don't have to change themselves to keep up with your success, and they can gossip to all their friends about your failure. I am sure you know people just like this.

> **WARNING!**
> For these next tasks you *must* ensure you have the appropriate space and uninterrupted, distraction-free environment to complete them. The findings may be confronting and challenging for you, but they are necessary to face head on. My advice is to not commence these tasks until you have the appropriate distraction-free environment to support the outcomes.

ACTION 28: IDENTIFYING OTHER PEOPLE'S LIMITING BELIEFS

Write down the names of all the people in your life that you feel place their limiting beliefs on you.

_____

_____

_____

_____

_____

_____

ACTION 29: IDENTIFYING OTHER PEOPLE'S LIMITING BELIEFS

Next to each person, write down what those people say or do to have a negative impact on you. Write down why you think they say and do these things.

_____

_____

_____

_____

_____

_____

_____

_____

ACTION 30: IDENTIFYING NEGATIVE INFLUENCES

Give each person a rating (1–10) of how much their words and actions affect you.
1 = rolls right off you and has no impact. 10 = makes you question everything.

_____

_____

_____

_____

_____

_____

_____

_____

Well done! If you've completed these tasks, this is a significant step in your transformational thinking. If you haven't done the tasks, then you need to STOP now and not go any further in this book until you have completed them.

The final step in this process is determining what you are now going to do about it. This can be tricky to navigate, but if you follow the guidelines below, it will put you in a good place to make the right decision for you.

ACTION 31: BUILDING YOUR EMOTIONAL FITNESS

Taking into consideration the tasks above, I want you to take 5–10 minutes to write down all the emotions you feel when you think about these negative people in your life. Reflect deeply and let the feelings come to you.

_____

_____

_____

_____

_____

_____

Now it's time to act in response to these feelings. Sometimes in life, we must make tough decisions to take our life to the next level. That requires courage. You need to be bold and brave as we go into this next phase.

ACTION 32: CATEGORIES OF NEGATIVE INFLUENCES

For the people you have noted as being removed from your life, I want you to now categorize those people falling into the following:

A. **No-Fuss Elimination**. These people can be easily eliminated from your life with no consequences (e.g., deleting a friend on Facebook).

B. **On-Watch Elimination**. If these people modify their behavior, you'll be happy to keep them in your life.

C. **Stuck with Them**. These people will always be a part of your life, no matter how they behave (e.g., parents, siblings).

Category A: No-Fuss Elimination

The people falling into category A could be "friends" on Facebook or other social media outlets that you can simply "unfriend" without consequence. Maybe it's someone you see from time to time through your group of friends that you could intentionally see less often without anyone noticing. You don't have to do it horribly, but remember that life is short, and you only want to surround yourself with quality people who lift you up. There comes a time when enough is enough and you need to make a change, and unfortunately, this includes drawing some lines around who you spend time with.

Write down those people you identified in action 32 who fall into this category that you can eliminate from your life with no fuss.

Category B: On-Watch Elimination

The people falling into category B can be tough to deal with. People in this category could be adding value to your life, but you believe they need to modify their behavior to be an effective support system for you. This requires a heartfelt conversation with the relevant individuals to express how you feel and explain the impact the relationship is having on you.

Sometimes, people are aware of their influence, but much of the time, they're not. My advice is to create a plan for these talks. Make some notes detailing what you'd like the outcome of your discussion to be. Is it to end the relationship, or is it to have them modify their behavior? Do you also need to modify your behavior? What does that look like to you? Is it an easy fix that can occur by the end of the conversation, or is it something that will take time? What could you do differently in your behavior to achieve the outcome you desire?

They may not take your feedback well, especially if they feel attacked. So, don't go in swinging. Let it be an honest conversation. And if they're unaware of the negative impact their words can have on you, they may be more likely than you think to want to change and to want to help. Give the people in your life the opportunity to show their love and support before eliminating them from your life.

Write down those people you identified in action 32 who fall into this category.

_____

_____

_____

_____

_____

Category C: Stuck with Them

People falling into category C will generally be your family, parents, siblings, and extended relatives. You didn't pick them, and you are stuck with them! These people have the potential to bring amazing gifts into your life, but at the same time, they can be destructive—if you let them.

Chances are these people will be in your life for a very long time. How to manage them is mostly the same as for those in category B. Your family can be incredibly rewarding, but it can also be the most damaging, so it is crucial to have frank conversations and resolve the issues that upset you. Resolution for you could simply be not spending as much time with them or no longer catching up with them. The choice is yours.

Write down those people you identified in action 32 who fall into this category and who will continue to be a part of your life forever.

_____

_____

_____

_____

_____

ACTION 33: ELIMINATING NEGATIVE INFLUENCES

Take 3 minutes and write down those people that you would greatly benefit from either eliminating from your life or at least dramatically reducing the time you spend with them.

Next to each person, write down the emotions you would experience once you've made that decision and the empowering significance that this will have on your life.

I know how difficult it can be to make change. I've personally made significant changes in my own life that I pondered for years before making the decisions that would change my life forever. Most significant was the decision to leave my marriage and 20-year relationship with my ex-wife. I'm not suggesting that you end marriages and long-term relationship on a whim. In fact, I believe that most people don't work hard enough on their intimate relationships prior to giving up and walking away. What I am suggesting is that you need to reflect deeply upon your existing relationships and act in a way that supports and nurtures you to become a better version of yourself for you and all of those who you want to empower in your beautiful life.

_____

_____

_____

_____

_____

ACTION 34: TAKING THE OTHER PERSON'S PERSPECTIVE

Before having conversations with anyone, take the time to put yourself in the other person's shoes. You must write down your answers to the following questions to properly prepare for the upcoming discussion. I understand that most of us do not like conflict or potential conflict discussions. They can be uncomfortable. But remember that they are necessary. Before you go into these discussions, it is crucial that you prepare so that you address the concerns with logic and clear thinking instead of pure emotion. Consider each question below carefully, write your responses, and don't skip any of them! Don't forget, there are two people to consider (you and the other person) and these questions may prompt you to question how you view the current situation. Go for it!

How would I feel if this person spoke to me in the way I am going to speak to them (e.g., discussion points, the tone of my voice, the words I use)?

_____

_____

Is there a possibility that there is something going on in their life now that may be causing them to react or behave the way in which they are currently?

_____

_____

Am I only looking at the downside of the relationship and not considering the upside?

_____

_____

What am I grateful for in this relationship?

_____

_____

How can I best phrase the words to deliver the message in a way that I would appreciate if it was being said to me?

_____

_____

Am I being reasonable and rational about my feelings toward this person's behavior?

_____

_____

Am I being emotional and irrational about my feelings toward this person's behavior?

_____

_____

Where is the best environment to have this discussion?

_____

_____

When is the best time to have this discussion?

_____

_____

Remember that this is action to take your life to a new level. It requires work on your part to achieve this. Prepare your plan for these conversations by writing down notes. You could even bring them along if it would help. If nothing else, the person will hopefully appreciate the work you have put into the issue and will recognize its importance to you. Be under no illusion. What I ask of you is not for the fainthearted or something that most people would do. But we have established already that you're not most people and that you're committed to this change. This is a *must*-do step, no matter how uncomfortable.

ACTION 35: ACT NOW!

Once you've completed the above tasks, it's time to act. Contact each person and make a time to have the discussion. This can be over the phone, but face to face is always better. Texts, emails, and voicemail messages are not appropriate for this step. You've got this!

ACTION 36: FOLLOW THROUGH

I've included this one to state the obvious. Make sure you follow through by turning up to your arranged meeting and completing the discussion. Don't back out at the last minute because you're afraid. Don't back down or stray from your plan in the middle of the conversation.

Remember, this is something you believe is necessary for you to move your life and relationships to a new level. People don't like conflict, and I'm sure that's true for you too. Delivering your feelings in a heartfelt way is the best approach. Have faith in yourself. Have courage, and be brave. Act, and follow through.

ACTION 37: FOLLOW UP

Once you have completed all the above tasks, including having had all the discussions you need, write down the emotions you now feel. Do you feel empowered? Relieved?

Write down at least three positive emotions you feel as a result of having completed these exercises.

_____

_____

_____

_____

_____

_____

Limits Imposed by Injury or Illness

Most clients that I work with have an injury of some kind—minor soft tissue injuries, arthritis, osteoporosis, diabetes, heart disease, cancer, broken bones, torn ligaments, damaged muscles and tendons, no cartilage in knees, broken necks, broken toes, broken legs, broken ankles, brain injuries, mental health issues such as stress, anxiety depression, high blood pressure, heart disease, cancer, fibromyalgia, type 1 and 2 diabetes, and terminal conditions. You name it, I've seen it.

What's fantastic is that all of the clients I've seen with these conditions had one thing in common: the burning desire to still improve themselves physically. They're not giving up. They want to make change despite their existing conditions.

Some people reach out, telling me they would like to get healthier, but they're not sure if they can, because they have injuries or conditions. I tell everyone the same thing: We focus on what they can do rather than what they cannot.

Does this mean that exercise will require a little more care and expert guidance? Absolutely. It is critical to work safely and sustainably to lessen the impact of an injury or illness rather than exacerbate it. That's where qualified professionals and listening to your body come in.

Injuries, however, don't always mean that you are hindered from exercise at all. For instance, I have worked with many clients who tell me they have "bad knees" and can't do squats. They are often extremely overweight and don't do any exercise apart from walking. They think that's all they're able to do, given the pain that things like squats bring, but there are a couple of fundamental things that will help.

First, reducing their fat levels and body weight will reduce the pressure on their knees. Just imagine if you had to carry an extra 45 pounds (20 kilograms) or more around with you every day. It's going to take its toll on your joints. Healthy eating is key here and can enable better exercise.

Second, by strengthening the quadriceps (the front top of the thigh) and hamstring (the back of the thigh), we make the muscles stronger, placing more of the body's load through the muscle instead of the joint. These two factors combined have resulted in many of my clients either being pain free or, at a minimum, reaching significantly reduced levels of pain.

By doing nothing in this instance, life can feel "over" as far as health and fitness is concerned. You can't see a path forward that doesn't cause pain or further an injury. But the right advice and health and fitness plan can make you feel 100% empowered, capable, and unstoppable.

By way of another example, I'd like to share my personal experience with a shoulder injury. At the time of writing this book, I have been exercising for over 30 years, performing heavy powerlifting moves, such as bench presses, squats, and deadlifts. They can place a huge load on your body. From time to time, I would feel pain in the front part of my shoulder. I managed it with stretching, ice, and massage, but after a while, the pain became more frequent.

I began seeing a physiotherapist, who gave me specialized exercises for about 4 months in order to rehabilitate the injury. When I still wasn't seeing improvement, she sent me for an ultrasound. The resulting scan showed that I had a condition known as tendinosis, a condition that causes a thinning in the tendon. It essentially meant that if I kept pushing my shoulder, the tendon could rupture, resulting in surgery and possibly the end of heavy weightlifting.

I had already backed off my training over the previous 10 months by not doing any upper-body work to completely rest my shoulder. The way my body was changing weighed on my mind. Weight training was such a massive part of my life, and I didn't want to have to back away from it. But I also didn't want to end up in a position where I was unable to lift weights properly ever again. This diagnosis created a fear in me that I would be placing myself at risk of injury if I continued to push myself.

Eventually, I was referred to a sports medicine specialist, who prescribed anti-inflammatory medicine for me. For the first few weeks, I felt great! I was cured, I thought. But, as before, the pain came back again. I was back in the doctor's office until I was referred to yet another specialist for more testing.

An MRI later, the doctor explained that he could see I had a small osteophyte at the bottom of my shoulder that would cause me pain every time I lifted my arm above my head. Imagine a bony spur sticking out of the bottom of your shoulder. When you push upward, that spur pushes into a tendon or nerve, causing pain. He told me that no amount of physiotherapy was ever going to fix this problem, because there was a physical impingement causing the pain. This meant that my options were to deal with the pain or to undergo surgery.

I chose surgery. My doctor was confident I would make a full recovery and be able to continue with weightlifting absolutely pain free! It was music to my ears.

The surgery was a success. The doctor removed the small osteophyte, and after a few months of gradual recovery, I was back where I wanted to be.

Weightlifting remains such an important part of my life that it was a no-brainer to me to continue searching for answers rather than simply accepting my injury as part of life. It would have been easier to accept the first diagnosis of tendinosis than it was to explore all the possible solutions. I didn't have to go forward with all the tests that were offered. In fact, I didn't have to see a doctor at all. But I chose to because I wanted a different outcome. I have spoken with many clients who, upon feeling pain, just stop doing the painful activity altogether without seeking professional help. They give up and believe that this is just the way things are going to be now.

The point of sharing this story is to help you recognize that injuries happen. Diagnoses aren't always quick and accurate. But if you are committed to your journey, you cannot think of injuries as a barrier to success. You will need to be your own advocate and seek out professional help if you encounter pain. And if the pain continues, keep working with professionals, ask for referrals to different kinds of doctors, keep seeking a solution that works, and keep focusing on what you can do and not on what you can't. Just because one person tells you one thing about your injury, don't be afraid to ask for a second, third, or fourth opinion if they don't make sense to you. It's your body. It's your life.

DO NOT MOVE ON TO THE NEXT CHAPTER UNTIL YOU HAVE COMPLETED EVERY ACTION ITEM ABOVE. NO EXCUSES!

Summary

- There can be obstacles in our way that prevent us from truly awakening the sexy within.
- Obstacles come from our limiting beliefs, values, and past experiences.
- Obstacles can also come from the limiting beliefs, values, and past experiences of others.
- Injuries are not a death sentence. Focus on what you can do rather than what you cannot.
- It is possible to overcome all obstacles with courage, focus, and consistent action.

SUCCESS STORY:
Alex Campbell, 23 years old

In 12 weeks, Alex lost 38.5 pounds (18.8% weight loss), reduced his body fat by 9.4%, and lost a total of 28 inches off his chest, waist, hips, legs, and arms.

"Training with Robb has been amazing. I could not have achieved these results without him. He is friendly, motivating, and encouraging and has insight and knowledge as to how best to achieve the weight loss. I weighed 229 pounds when I first met Robb and now am currently 190.5 pounds.

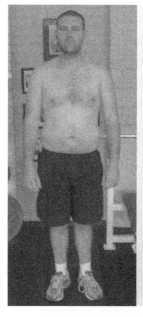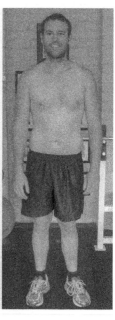

"My advice to anyone considering weight loss is, if you are 100% committed to losing weight once and for all, follow Robb's program. The nutrition plan is straightforward and easy to maintain, with enjoyable foods. I never really felt I was dieting, just eating healthily. The workouts are fantastic. Training with him has been great, and I always feel I'm getting an awesome workout. My before and after photos just seem unreal, and this was in just 12 weeks! I'm looking forward to continuing my training with Robb so we can reach my goal weight of 174 pounds. My lifestyle has changed noticeably, and I feel like I am a different person. I'm more confident, feeling happy, and enjoying everyday life!"

CHAPTER 5

Prepare to Be Sexy

As we get closer to performing the workouts, it is important to remind ourselves that sexiness is a journey, not a destination. There is no single workout, performed once, that will make you feel sexy. Never forget that optimizing your health and fitness is a lifelong journey. If you approach these upcoming workouts knowing that we are on a journey together to unveil the sexy you, then you're going to get the most value from them.

I have designed 52 workouts for you to complete. Some workouts require no equipment; others may require resistance bands or dumbbells. They have been specifically designed so that you don't have to join a gym if you don't want to. There's no need to invest in expensive equipment. You can find any of the equipment I've included in the workouts for just a few dollars if you shop online or ask around to some friends. (You'll be surprised how many sets of unused equipment are gathering dust and how happy people are to give them to you.)

So why 52 workouts? My intention has been to overdeliver to you a variety of workouts so that you remain inspired and motivated to achieve your sexiness. You may want to think about it as one new workout per week. Shortly, I will show you how you can even break these workouts down into shorter workouts and could create 156 workouts or more from the 52 included in *Awaken the Sexy within*. You are limited only by your imagination as to how to work with these 52

103

workouts into your schedule. To help you get started, I've outlined some examples of program planning cycles to choose from.

Recall from chapter 1 that you must have a plan, or you are planning to fail. Of the thousands of people I have personally trained over the past 30 years, I would say 99.9% of them had little to no previous structured program with their exercise or nutrition prior to the commencing a program with me. They do a few sets and repetitions for arms, legs, chest, and abs; a bit of cardio; and then the workout is over. They don't have a properly designed program written down to follow during a workout, and they aren't recording or tracking what they're doing during the workout.

Success must start with the end in mind. For instance, are you using these 52 workouts to supplement other training you're doing? Are you the type of person who gets bored easily? Do you work out best when your program remains unchanged for a period of weeks? Do you need to break your sessions up so that they're 20–30 min, rather than 45–60 min? Will you be exercising by yourself or with another person or people? Have you always tried to avoid cardio exercise?

You can map out your entire year of training if that is your preference, or you can break it down into smaller, manageable blocks.

Generally, most programs I design for clients are based around the following principles:

- 3–4 days per week of resistance training (e.g., lifting weights or body-weight exercises)
- 3–4 days per week of cardio training (e.g., walking, running, bicycling, swimming)

This frequency is what's needed to get you the sexiest possible results. But I also follow this principle: If you usually lead a sedentary lifestyle and you now aim to do just one workout per week, it is still better than before. It is certainly a step in the right direction. It's like climbing a set of stairs. If you want to get from the bottom of the stairs to the top, you don't have to do that in one step. You take one consistent step at a time, and you will get to the top. You just have to get started.

How to work out where you start may seem a little overwhelming at first, but follow my guidance principles below to help you:

1. ***Routine is crucial.*** Humans love an environment of structure and consistency to progress in life. Progress is critical for us to succeed. You must plan your week with this routine in mind. Scheduling the days you will train, the length of workouts, and the time of day you train will help create a successful mindset.

2. ***Know your current fitness levels.*** Make sure you have a pretty good handle on your current level of fitness. If you've never worked out and have 100 pounds or more to lose, it's best for you to start off slowly, with our beginner program. This is about you striving to achieve a sexy version of your body, not someone else's. You can progress and increase your intensity as you move through each workout and want to move to the next intermediate level of our programs. If you don't ever make it to the advanced levels, that's okay. You need to build progression slowly to help you stay motivated and prevent injury.

3. ***Allocate and schedule the time***. How much time are you going to allocate to your sexiness each week? I need you to think about this in terms of minutes and hours. Everyone I meet has a very hectic lifestyle. It is very easy for all of us to fill our days with tasks that need to be completed or watch the evening disappear by spending time on social media or watching television. But it comes down to priorities. My highest value in life is my health and fitness. I *make* the time for my workouts. For you to be successful in your sexiness journey, you need to make this a priority and schedule it. Otherwise, it won't happen by itself.

    Start with how long you want to work out for each session. What is important is to move more. I want you to move every single day. My aim for you is to be getting to the stage where you can do three to four of our workouts per week. But, as I mentioned above, if doing just one of the 52 workouts per week is enough for you to start with, I want you to at least walk every other day in accordance with the programming I've outlined at table 5.1. You build to two, three, and four workouts over time. Using the principles I have just mentioned, here is what a typical week in your schedule could look like:

Table 5.1. A Typical Week's Workout Program

Day	Workout Description
Monday	Resistance workout (refer to chapter 6, 15–60 min)
Tuesday	Cardio workout (e.g., walking for 10–40 min)
Wednesday	Resistance workout (refer to chapter 6, 15–60 min)
Thursday	Cardio workout (e.g., walking for 10–40 min)
Friday	Resistance workout (refer to chapter 6, 15–60 min)
Saturday	Cardio workout (e.g., walking for 10–40 min)
Sunday	Cardio workout (e.g., walking for 10–40 min)

If exercise is not currently a part of your every day life, you need to rate your awakening of sexiness as a much higher priority in your life than it is currently. You may not think you have any further time in your day to devote to exercise, but I challenge anyone to not find a way to at least fit in 10–30 minutes of exercise every single day. This is *your* sexiness mission. It comes down to your priorities and how badly you want it.

Here's some strategies that work well to make the time:

- Get out of bed, and start your day 30–60 minutes earlier. If you think getting up at 6:00 a.m. is hard, I start my day at 4:20 a.m. and get 3–4 hours of work done before most people start their day. If I can do it, I'm sure you can set the alarm a few minutes earlier to focus on your health.
- Go to bed 30–60 minutes later and exercise in the evening.
- Make time during your lunch break to exercise.
- Reduce the amount of time you watch television.
- Reduce the amount of time you spend on social media.
- Break your sessions into smaller, bite-size pieces, such as 10-minute mini sessions, as opposed to missing a session altogether.

- Look through your existing schedule with a view that you absolutely MUST find and schedule the time you need for you to achieve your sexiness.
- Don't settle for less than you deserve.
- Don't make excuses.
- Don't keep sacrificing your needs for everyone else around you.
- Make a way to have all that you need to awaken the sexy within!

4. *Track your progress.* It doesn't matter where you start, as long as you keep moving forward to the next stage. I've worked with clients that find it difficult to walk to their mailbox and back once per day. That's okay. It's a start. The next day, I ask them to do that again, then try twice per day, then the next day, twice per day again, then three times per day, then 100 yards more, to the end of their block, then around the block. Get the idea?

5. *Manage intensity.* There are two big reasons for failure. Going too hard too fast can cause burnout and injury. Not working hard enough doesn't yield results. You should be working out at an intensity such that you can still carry out a conversation, but you feel your breathing level has elevated. As a generally acceptable guide for fat burning, I use the following formula:

180 beats per minute (bpm) – your age = your fat-burning zone

Your fat-burning zone is the intensity level that will help you burn the most fat. When you exercise at a higher intensity, your body will seek out energy that is most easily accessible. This mostly means seeking energy from food. When you exercise at a moderate intensity, or within your fat-burning zone, your body doesn't need as much energy instantly, so instead, it sources the energy primarily from fat.

ACTION 38: CALCULATING YOUR FAT-BURNING ZONE

Calculate your own fat-burning range using the formula above. If you are 40 years old, your fat-burning zone will be 140 (180 minus 40), for example.

My point here is to measure your effort and use your heart rate as a general guide. You can purchase an effective and economical heart rate monitor that will give you a reasonably accurate measurement of your heart rate while you're working out. After you have been using one for a while, you will gain a good understanding of how hard you need to work to stay in your target heart rate zone. You'll feel it in your body. I personally know when my heart rate gets to 142 bpm, as I can start to hear my heart beating in my eardrums. You'll develop your own level of awareness.

Below, I've mapped out some examples of 8-week programs you can use for the workouts I've provided. Note that each of these workouts is designed to be approximately 60 minutes in length if the workout is completed as it is written. As I've noted up to this point, if you feel this is not within your capabilities to begin with, here are a few tips for you to modify the workout to suit you:

- Reduce the workout by decreasing the number of sets that need to be completed.
- Reduce the number of repetitions.
- Reduce the time of each round for those rounds based on timing. For example, if the workout prescribes 60 seconds, cut it down to 45 or 30 seconds.
- Start at the beginning of the workout, and complete as much as you feel capable of before stopping. For instance, if you can only manage 10 minutes of workout time when you're first starting out, then stop at that point. Track and challenge yourself to progress when you feel able.

FITNESS ASSESSMENT

What gets measured gets done! I've mentioned it before, and I will keep saying it. Measuring and tracking your progress are essential for you to awaken the sexy within. Read chapter 3, on accountability, again. You will be seven to eight times more likely to succeed if you track what it is that you are doing with your health and fitness. Most clients I work with are looking to shed several pounds of fat. I've worked with people wanting to gain 20 pounds (10 kilograms) of muscle through to those who want to lose 250 pounds (120 kilograms) of fat. It really doesn't matter where you are right now. The point is that we need to measure exactly where you are now, then measure your progress against that initial assessment.

Most people only measure their success based on the number they see on the scales. The problem with this approach is that it doesn't consider progress you have been making in other areas. Your body is composed of water, muscle, and fat. Right now, you will weigh a certain weight. Let's say, for example, that you currently weigh 175 pounds (80 kilograms). At that weight, you will have a certain body fat percentage. Let's now say that after 4 weeks of following your meal plan and exercise program, you stand on the scales and there is no change in your weight. You're okay with the results, but you really wanted at least 4–8 pounds (2–4 kilograms) of weight loss. Does that mean you've been unsuccessful? I would say the answer is yes—if you are only focused on what the scales show you.

However, if you complete the fitness assessment below, you will see that the number on the scales is merely one component of success. The reality could be that your measurements have reduced, that you've put on 4 pounds of muscle and lost 4 pounds of fat. It's just that the scales reflect no downward movement, but your body fat percentage has improved. You feel great, you're sleeping better, you're functionally stronger, and you have more energy. Now, that sounds much more powerful than no change in the scales, don't you think? Therefore, it is so important to capture this data when you first begin. The ongoing assessments will go a long way to keeping you inspired and motivated.

ACTION 39: TAKE YOUR FIRST FITNESS ASSESSMENT

It's time! Here are the steps to completing your fitness assessment. I suggest you complete a fitness assessment every 4 weeks to keep you on track.

Step 1: Print Out the Assessment

Even though the fitness assessment is included below, print off additional copies of the fitness assessment document at AwakenTheSexyWithin.com. Complete the fitness assessment at a time of day that is convenient for you, and use the same time of day each time you complete it. Ensure you complete the assessment after you are properly warmed up and have at least had a light, nutritious snack from your meal plan prior to beginning it.

Step 2: See Your Doctor

Unless you've done this in the past 3 months, make an appointment with your doctor for an annual physical. Depending on your medical history, I suggest that you have this checkup at least once per year or as otherwise required by your doctor or specialist.

I suggest you have the following tested:

- Blood test: cholesterol
- Blood test: liver function
- Blood test: iron levels
- Blood test: diabetes test
- Women over 20: pap smear to test for cervical cancer
- Women over 40: mammogram to test for breast cancer
- Men and women over 50: test for bowel cancer
- Men over 50: blood test PSA to test for prostate cancer
- Men and women: skin check for skin cancer
- Men and women: blood pressure

Step 3: Take Your Measurements

Use a dressmaker's measuring tape wrapped around each body part listed here:

- Bicep: center of the biceps while flexed.
- Chest: center line of chest. Breathe in deeply and take the measurement after the exhale.
- Waist: On your belly button or narrowest part of your waist, take the measurement when your belly is sucked in as far as possible. The reason I measure this way is that the temptation from people in the second fitness assessment is to always suck in their tummy! If we do this on the first assessment, you will be consistent.
- Hips: center of the buttocks.
- Thighs: standing up tall with level shoulders and hands down by your sides, fingers curled up (like a fist), thumb pointing down, measured at the point at the bottom of the thumb.
- Calves: center of the calf muscle.

Be sure to measure in the center of the muscle and, preferably, have someone else take your measurements on your behalf. If you do have someone else take the measurements, ensure that you use the same person each time. Add your measurements to your printed fitness assessment sheet.

Step 4: Weigh Yourself

Stand on a scale, and record your weight. For the best results, I suggest always using the same time of day and the same scales. After getting up and using the restroom, weigh yourself without any clothes on.

It's important for women to note that you will be more fluid retentive during your monthly menstrual cycle, which can cause fluctuations in weight. To keep your results consistent, steer clear of the fitness assessment at that time and capture your weight mid-cycle instead. Record your result on your fitness assessment sheet.

Step 5: Take Some Photos

Before-and-after photos are crucial to tracking your progress and how far you've come. For women, I suggest using a two-piece bathing suit or bra and underwear. Men should wear only underwear or shorts but should stay away from long, baggy shorts. You need to be able to see as much skin as possible so that the changes will be very evident as you progress. Take a photo from all four sides—front, left side, right side, back. To do this well, I suggest asking someone that you trust to take them. Be sure to store your photos and results somewhere you can easily retrieve them as required.

Step 6: Warm-up

Perform a 5-minute warm-up after you have completed steps 1–4, as your measurements can vary between when you are cold and when you are warm or hot. Your warm-up could be as simple as walking around the block, riding a stationary bike, doing 5 minutes of vigorous housework, etc.

Step 7: The Strength Test

This section of the test is crucial to assess your level of strength across several different body parts. The aim is to complete as many repetitions as possible within 1 minute. You will need a stopwatch or countdown timer for this test. Please refer to the workout section of *Awaken the Sexy within* to ensure your form and technique are correct for each exercise:

- Sit-ups
- Power jacks

- Plank (maximum time you can hold this position)
- Push-ups
- Squats
- Dips
- Burpees
- Heel touches

Write down how you did on your fitness assessment sheet.

Step 8: The Cardio Test

This part of the assessment has a focus on your cardiovascular fitness. You need to pace yourself in this part of the test, because if you push too hard too soon, you may start to feel sick. The aim of this component of the test is to complete each of the seven exercises below, with as little rest as possible, until you are finished. Get a stopwatch out and time yourself; only stop the watch when you have completed all seven exercises. This test is challenging!

1. 250 climbers (each change of feet is one)
2. 15 sit-ups
3. 25 squat jumps
4. 25 push-ups
5. 15 sit-ups
6. 25 squat jumps
7. 250 climbers (each change of feet is one)

Write down your results on your fitness assessment sheet.

Step 9: Cool Down

As your heart rate comes down, do some simple stretches (examples can be found at AwakenTheSexyWithin.com).

Step 10: Analyze the Results

For your first fitness assessment, you can use the spaces below, but for future assessments, go to AwakenTheSexyWithin.com and print the successes and challenges worksheet.

Analyze your results and write down at least three successes and three challenges you have faced over the last 4 weeks.

_____

_____

_____

_____

_____

How would you rate your adherence and compliance with your nutrition plan and workouts over the past 4 weeks (scale of 1–10, with 10 representing 100% compliance)? Please write down why you have rated yourself with this score.

_____

_____

_____

Write down the improvement opportunities that exist for you.

_____

_____

_____

What are your goals for the next 4 weeks?

_____

_____

Use the rating table below to rate yourself against the fitness assessment results of others. This will help you determine which of the 9-week sample workout programs are suitable for you and the appropriate level of intensity to apply to each workout.

Fitness Assessment Rating Table

	Description	Beginner	Intermediate	Advanced
1	Sit-ups (AMRAP)	20	35	60+
2	Power jacks (AMRAP)	20	35	55+
3	Plank (maximum hold)	At least 30 sec	60–90 sec	Up to 2 min
4	Push-ups (AMRAP)	20	35	50+
5	Squats (AMRAP)	30	40	60+
6	Dips (AMRAP)	30	40	50+
7	Burpees (AMRAP)	10	10–20	20+
8	Heel touches (AMRAP)	80	120	175+
9	Cardiovascular fitness test	Up to 13 min	Up to 10 min	Up to 6 min
Note: AMRAP = As many repetitions as possible within 1 min				

Please be sure that you've completed the fitness assessment as outlined above before commencing your first workout. You must measure your progress and that will happen most effectively if you do the fitness assessment every 4 weeks, without exception. I can tell you that most people do not do this. They don't measure their progress. Chances are you haven't done this before either. This is one more element contributing to most people never achieving the ultimate sexy body they desire. I make no apologies for harping on this point. Follow what I say, and you will look back and see how crucial completing the fitness assessments on a consistent basis was in helping you track your progress and keeping you focused on your ultimate sexy body. Focus!

To make it easier for you to get started with your workouts, I've outlined below some sample 9-week plans, where I have laid out for you what to do on which days. Of course, you can just start at workout 1 and progress from there, but these plans make it very simple to get started without having to think about what to do and when. I've done the hard work for you. Based on the results of your fitness assessment, this will help you determine whether you should be starting with a beginner, intermediate, or advanced plan.

You can choose from the following:

- Sample beginner plan 1
- Sample beginner plan 2
- Sample intermediate plan 1
- Sample intermediate plan 2
- Sample advanced plan 1
- Sample advanced plan 2

SAMPLE BEGINNER PLAN 1

Week	Mon	Tues	Wed	Thurs	Fri	Sat	Sun
1	Fitness assessment	Cardio 1	Workout 1	Cardio 1	Workout 1	Cardio 1	Cardio 1
2	Workout 2	Cardio 1	Workout 3	Cardio 1	Workout 4	Cardio 1	Cardio 1
3	Workout 2	Cardio 1	Workout 3	Cardio 1	Workout 4	Cardio 1	Cardio 1
4	Workout 1	Cardio 1	Workout 1	Cardio 1	Workout 1	Cardio 1	Cardio 1
5	Fitness assessment	Cardio 2	Workout 5	Cardio 2	Workout 6	Cardio 2	Cardio 2
6	Workout 7	Cardio 2	Workout 8	Cardio 2	Workout 9	Cardio 2	Cardio 2
7	Workout 10	Cardio 2	Workout 11	Cardio 2	Workout 12	Cardio 2	Cardio 2
8	Workout 13	Cardio 2	Workout 14	Cardio 2	Workout 15	Cardio 2	Cardio 2
9	Fitness assessment	Cardio 2	Workout 16	Cardio 2	Workout 17	Cardio 2	Cardio 2

Cardio 1: During this phase, focus on walking or low-impact exercise, such as stationary bike riding, swimming, etc. Focus on moving within your fat-burning heart rate (as you calculated above as 180 bpm minus your age) for 10–20 minutes at a time.

Cardio 2: Focus on 15–20 minutes of cardio, as noted above, but you should now start to find that you can increase your intensity a little further as you now have some conditioning. Be sure to keep your heart rate in your fat-burning zone.

SAMPLE BEGINNER PLAN 2

Week	Mon	Tues	Wed	Thurs	Fri	Sat	Sun
1	Fitness assessment	Cardio 1	Workout 1	Cardio 1	Workout 2	Cardio 1	Cardio 1
2	Workout 3	Cardio 1	Workout 4	Cardio 1	Workout 5	Cardio 1	Cardio 1
3	Workout 6	Cardio 1	Workout 7	Cardio 1	Workout 8	Cardio 1	Cardio 1
4	Workout 9	Cardio 1	Workout 10	Cardio 1	Workout 11	Cardio 1	Cardio 1
5	Fitness assessment	Cardio 2	Workout 5	Cardio 2	Workout 6	Cardio 2	Cardio 2
6	Workout 12	Cardio 2	Workout 13	Cardio 2	Workout 14	Cardio 2	Cardio 2
7	Workout 15	Cardio 2	Workout 16	Cardio 2	Workout 17	Cardio 2	Cardio 2
8	Workout 18	Cardio 2	Workout 19	Cardio 2	Workout 20	Cardio 2	Cardio 2
9	Fitness assessment	Cardio 2	Workout 21	Cardio 2	Workout 22	Cardio 2	Cardio 2

Cardio 1: During this phase, focus on walking or low-impact exercise, such as stationary bike riding, swimming, etc. Focus on moving within your fat-burning heart rate (as you calculated above as 180 bpm minus your age) for 10–20 minutes of duration.

Cardio 2: Focus on 15–20 minutes of cardio, as noted above, but you should now start to find that you can increase your intensity a little further as you now have some conditioning. Be sure to keep your heart rate in the same fat-burning range of 180 bpm minus your age.

SAMPLE INTERMEDIATE PLAN 1

You will note that this program is the same as sample beginner plan 2; however, the difference is to graduate from the beginner section of the workout to the intermediate option. Where an intermediate option is not provided, look to raise your intensity level slightly from beginner level.

Week	Mon	Tues	Wed	Thurs	Fri	Sat	Sun
1	Fitness assessment	Cardio 1	Workout 1	Cardio 1	Workout 1	Cardio 1	Cardio 1
2	Workout 2	Cardio 1	Workout 3	Cardio 1	Workout 4	Cardio 1	Cardio 1
3	Workout 2	Cardio 1	Workout 3	Cardio 1	Workout 4	Cardio 1	Cardio 1
4	Workout 1	Cardio 1	Workout 1	Cardio 1	Workout 1	Cardio 1	Cardio 1
5	Fitness assessment	Cardio 2	Workout 5	Cardio 2	Workout 6	Cardio 2	Cardio 2
6	Workout 7	Cardio 2	Workout 8	Cardio 2	Workout 9	Cardio 2	Cardio 2
7	Workout 10	Cardio 2	Workout 11	Cardio 2	Workout 12	Cardio 2	Cardio 2
8	Workout 13	Cardio 2	Workout 14	Cardio 2	Workout 15	Cardio 2	Cardio 2
9	Fitness assessment	Cardio 2	Workout 16	Cardio 2	Workout 17	Cardio 2	Cardio 2

Cardio 1: During this phase, focus on walking or low-impact exercise, such as stationary bike riding, swimming, etc. Focus on moving within your fat-burning heart rate (as you calculated above as 180 bpm minus your age) for 20–30 minutes of duration.

SAMPLE INTERMEDIATE PLAN 2

Week	Mon	Tues	Wed	Thurs	Fri	Sat	Sun
1	Fitness assessment	Cardio 1	Workout 1	Cardio 1	Workout 2	Cardio 1	Cardio 1
2	Workout 3	Cardio 1	Workout 4	Cardio 1	Workout 5	Cardio 1	Cardio 1
3	Workout 6	Cardio 1	Workout 7	Cardio 1	Workout 8	Cardio 1	Cardio 1
4	Workout 9	Cardio 1	Workout 10	Cardio 1	Workout 11	Cardio 1	Cardio 1
5	Fitness assessment	Cardio 1	Workout 5	Cardio 1	Workout 6	Cardio 1	Cardio 1
6	Workout 12	Cardio 1	Workout 13	Cardio 1	Workout 14	Cardio 1	Cardio 1
7	Workout 15	Cardio 1	Workout 16	Cardio 1	Workout 17	Cardio 1	Cardio 1
8	Workout 18	Cardio 1	Workout 19	Cardio 1	Workout 20	Cardio 1	Cardio 1
9	Fitness assessment	Cardio 1	Workout 21	Cardio 1	Workout 22	Cardio 1	Cardio 1

Cardio 1: During this phase, focus on walking or low-impact exercise, such as stationary bike riding, swimming, etc. Focus on moving within your fat-burning heart rate (as you calculated above as 180 bpm minus your age) for 20–30 minutes of duration.

SAMPLE ADVANCED PLAN 1

You will note that this program is the same as the plan 2 samples for beginners and intermediate: however, the difference is to graduate from the intermediate section of the workout to the advanced option. Where an advanced option is not provided, look to raise your intensity level slightly from intermediate level.

Week	Mon	Tues	Wed	Thurs	Fri	Sat	Sun
1	Fitness assessment	Cardio 1	Workout 1	Cardio 1	Workout 1	Cardio 1	Cardio 1
2	Workout 2	Cardio 1	Workout 3	Cardio 1	Workout 4	Cardio 1	Cardio 1
3	Workout 2	Cardio 1	Workout 3	Cardio 1	Workout 4	Cardio 1	Cardio 1
4	Workout 1	Cardio 1	Workout 1	Cardio 1	Workout 1	Cardio 1	Cardio 1
5	Fitness assessment	Cardio 2	Workout 5	Cardio 2	Workout 6	Cardio 2	Cardio 2
6	Workout 7	Cardio 2	Workout 8	Cardio 2	Workout 9	Cardio 2	Cardio 2
7	Workout 10	Cardio 2	Workout 11	Cardio 2	Workout 12	Cardio 2	Cardio 2
8	Workout 13	Cardio 2	Workout 14	Cardio 2	Workout 15	Cardio 2	Cardio 2
9	Fitness assessment	Cardio 2	Workout 16	Cardio 2	Workout 17	Cardio 2	Cardio 2

Cardio 1: During this phase, focus on walking or low-impact exercise, such as stationary bike riding, swimming, etc. Focus on moving within your fat-burning heart rate (as you calculated above as 180bpm minus your age) for 20–40 minutes.

SAMPLE ADVANCED PLAN 2

Week	Mon	Tues	Wed	Thurs	Fri	Sat	Sun
1	Fitness assessment	Cardio 1	Workout 1	Cardio 1	Workout 1	Cardio 1	Cardio 1
2	Workout 2	Cardio 1	Workout 52	Cardio 1	Workout 3	Cardio 1	Cardio 1
3	Workout 4	Cardio 1	Workout 49	Cardio 1	Workout 5	Cardio 1	Cardio 1
4	Workout 11	Cardio 1	Workout 46	Cardio 1	Workout 14	Cardio 1	Cardio 1
5	Fitness assessment	Cardio 2	Workout 40	Cardio 2	Workout 6	Cardio 2	Cardio 2
6	Workout 7	Cardio 2	Workout 36	Cardio 2	Workout 8	Cardio 2	Cardio 2
7	Workout 9	Cardio 2	Workout 27	Cardio 2	Workout 10	Cardio 2	Cardio 2
8	Workout 11	Cardio 2	Workout 14	Cardio 2	Workout 12	Cardio 2	Cardio 2
9	Fitness assessment	Cardio 2	Workout 16	Cardio 2	Workout 17	Cardio 2	Cardio 2

9 Ways to Mix Up Your Workout Programs

1. Start at workout 1, and select one new workout to perform each week For example, week 1 could be workout 1, week 2 could be workout 2, and week 3 could be workout 3.

2. As above, but start at workout 52 and work backward.

3. As above, but select random numbers between 1 and 52 to select each workout. Without doubling up on the same workout, continue workouts until you've completed all 52.

4. Read through each workout and find the top 12 workouts that are most appealing to you. Use these 12 workouts as the basis of the next 5 weeks of your training, ensuring you don't double-up on the workout.

5. Review each workout, and identify those that you feel will be the most challenging for you. Make sure you do at least one of these workouts each week.

6. Review the index and details of each workout, and select the body part you would like to have as your focus for the workout. For example, sexy

legs 1 has a prime focus of working your legs from many different angles to stimulate muscle growth and toning.

7. If you're just getting started with working out, review the first 12 workouts and select those workouts you believe will be most manageable for you. Stick to these workouts for the first 5 weeks before graduating to workouts you believe to be more challenging for you.

8. Select at least one workout per week you could do with a buddy or partner and have them join you for the workout.

9. Plan your entire year of workouts in 12 4-week blocks. Be creative, using the above tips 1–9, and make each 4-week block different. For example, weeks 1–4 could be workouts 1–12, week 5–8 could be random workouts from 1 to 52, weeks 9–12 could be 12 of your favorite workouts, etc.

Important Facts before You Start Your Workout

1. Make sure you've created your workout plan from earlier in this chapter and have this printed out and on display somewhere prominent in your home or workspace. You need to be able to refer to it each day. I suggest you tick or cross off each workout and cardio session as you do it. That helps create momentum for you to ensure you keep progressing toward your goal.

2. Choose an appropriate day and time for your workouts so that you establish a routine for success. Block that time out in your schedule. I personally use Google calendar; other people find a manual diary works for them. Whatever the mechanism, block it out, and stick to it!

3. Ensure your environment is right for your workout. Take into consideration the climate (e.g., is it too cold or too hot?). Do you have enough space for your workout? Do you prefer working out inside or outside?

4. Review the equipment needed for each exercise on your plan at the start of each week. If you do not have the items needed, consider purchasing them, finding something similar around your home, or selecting a different workout. Don't wait until it's time to start the workout to realize you are missing something. You'll be much more likely to skip it entirely if you do.

5. Make sure you have drinking water available and the type of music that will inspire and motivate you to have a great workout. Create some awesome workout playlists throughout the week so you don't have to worry about creating them during the workout.

6. Have your phone or a stopwatch available for the workouts that require timed intervals. For the workouts involving Tabata training (e.g., 20 seconds of working time, 10 seconds of rest), there are many free Tabata apps available, so be sure to download one prior to your workout.

7. Pace yourself through the workouts, especially if this is the first workout you've ever undertaken or if you haven't exercised in a long time. If you push too hard too quickly, you are placing yourself in a higher risk category to have injuries. Listen to your body, and respond accordingly. You've got your entire life ahead of you. There's no need to push yourself beyond your limits. Start out slowly, and build up the intensity of the sessions as your strength and fitness levels improve.

8. Delayed onset of muscle soreness (DOMS) is real and can hit your body hard. Sometimes, when I do a workout and push very hard, I can feel sore by the end of the workout. What I know is that 24 hours later, I will feel even more sore. In 48 hours, I will be the sorest. After 48 hours, the muscles generally begin to recover, and the soreness dissipates. If you are a beginner or haven't worked out for a while, realize that this will most likely be your fate for the first few sessions as your body experiences the changes you are subjecting it to. Just remember that it is all normal. Follow the stretching programming at the end of each workout, and stretch a few more times throughout the day as you need it. Keep in mind that getting the blood circulating through to the sore muscles is the best way to help them recover. That means being active. I suggest a 20–30 minute walk each day to help you recover faster.

   There is also a difference between good pain and bad pain. Good pain is muscle soreness. Bad pain is the pain you feel in the joint. If you're feeling pain in your muscles, that is normal. Pain in the joint is something we want to avoid, so if the pain persists, double-check your technique, modify your exercise, and, if the pain persists, seek the help of a medical professional. Don't forget what you learned in chapter 4: There is always an alternate approach to achieving the outcome you desire.

9. Drink your 50+ fluid ounces of water per day in between your workouts, as this will not only keep you hydrated but will also help flush out the toxins from your sore muscles and greatly speed up the recovery process.

10. Each exercise allocated in the workouts is accompanied by a photo and description explaining how the exercise is to be performed. I suggest familiarizing yourself with the exercises prior to commencing the workout, so you can complete it with as little disruption as possible. Refer to AwakenTheSexyWithin.com for a full list of all the exercises.

11. Track your workout completion by marking it off your printed 9-week plan template.

12. Have fun! After all, these workouts are going to awaken the sexy within you! Visualize each workout taking you one step closer to your sexiness. Focus!

DO NOT MOVE ON TO THE NEXT CHAPTER UNTIL YOU HAVE COMPLETED EVERY ACTION ITEM ABOVE. NO EXCUSES!

Summary

- Obtain clearance from the appropriate health professionals that you are okay to commence working out.
- Select or create your workout plan for the next 9 weeks.
- Complete the fitness assessment every 4 weeks, starting at week 0.
- Create a schedule for the days and times of each workout, and ensure you adhere to it.
- Exercise in an appropriate, empowering environment.
- Ensure you have the appropriate equipment you need, including a timer, stopwatch, and relevant apps.
- Have drinking water and motivational music on hand for each workout.
- Listen to your body, and pace yourself through each workout.
- Be aware of DOMS, drink 50+ fluid ounces of water per day, and stay active, with walking for at least 20–30 minutes per day.

- Check AwakenTheSexyWithin.com to understand how each exercise is performed correctly.
- Track your completion of each workout.
- Challenge yourself with each workout.
- While you're warming up for each workout, take that time to focus on what you are about to do, and connect each workout with your goal of awakening your own sexy within.

SUCCESS STORY:
Lisa Braaksma, 41 years old

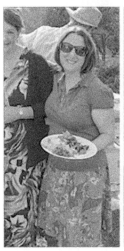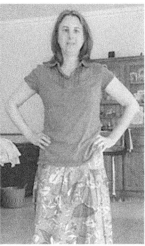

Lisa has lost 42 pounds and had a dramatic reduction in body fat and lost inches from her entire body. Lisa has had an awesome increase in her fitness and now has more energy to chase after her seven children! Lisa's incredible transformation also includes improving her eating habits and dramatically improved strength.

Fast track 3 years later, and Lisa was involved in a serious car accident. She hit a tree that lay across the road after being brought down by a storm, travelling at 55 mph late at night.

As you can see from the x-ray in the photo, Lisa broke her C2 vertebra and was unable to move without pain for many months. In fact, she almost lost her life.

Lisa's never-give-up attitude and drive to get back into her training after rehabilitation and become functionally strong again have been inspirational.

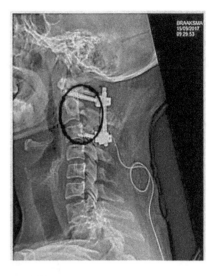

"I was told I was very fortunate not to have become a paraplegic in my accident, but after month 6 of my recovery, I came to realize what NO EXERCISE can do to one's body. I was still eating healthy and keeping up with Robb's meal plan, but my clothes were getting tight, and the scales were climbing! Not being able to exercise was incredibly frustrating. After 3 months, I was attending physiotherapy and was given minor exercises to strengthen my neck, but they didn't focus on the areas where I wanted to lose fat.

"After 8 months, I was given the green light to start doing weight training with Robb. I am so grateful for the strength I built prior to the accident, as this has made my recovery faster and provided me with essential mobility. I am getting stronger every day, thanks to the work with Robb and physiotherapy. I am still alive AND determined to get my body, strength, and fitness back to where I was before my accident, then make it better than ever! Thank you, Robb. I couldn't have done this without you."

CHAPTER 6

Work Your Way to Sexy

Workout Name	Workout Name
1. Total-body classic	27. OMG no more squats please
2. Tabata town 1	28. Pack of cards 2
3. Sweat 99 to 1	29. Climbing superset 2
4. Sexy legs 1	30. Leg smasher
5. The road to hell and back	31. Circuit intensity 1
6. Pack of cards 1	32. Tabata town 3
7. Partner smasher 1	33. The 48s
8. Climbing superset 1	34. Boxing body tone 1
9. The dirty dozen	35. Quads on fire
10. Four rounds to hell 1	36. Exhaustion workout 1
11. Killer 90–50, 50–90	37. Buns of Steel
12. Partner smasher 2	38. AMRAP madness 3
13. Abs and HIIT smasher	39. Climbing superset 3
14. Total body ab blaster 1	40. Tabata town 4
15. Max overload 1	41. Total-body ab blaster 3
16. AMRAP madness 1	42. Jumping 40s
17. Six-packs and guns	43. Beach legs
18. 1,000 reps	44. Boxing body tone 2
19. Sweat It Out—10 to 1	45. Circuit intensity 2
20. Partner ladder reps	46. Pack of Cards 3
21. Pyramids and mountains	47. Three to thrive
22. Exploding 50s	48. Let's work it
23. Tabata town 2	49. Four rounds to hell 3
24. Four rounds to hell 2	50. Sneaky
25. Total-body ab blaster 2	51. Magnificent seven
26. AMRAP madness 2	52. Pyramids in Japan

Workout 1: Total-Body Classic

Warm-up

Your 5-minute warm-up could be as simple as walking around the block, riding a stationary bike, doing 5 minutes of vigorous housework, etc. The important point is to ensure you are appropriately warmed up before performing any of the exercises.

Workout

This is a great whole-body workout and can be performed with body-weighted exercises, kettlebells (KB), resistance bands (RB), dumbbells, or a combination of all four. It's a classic workout, because it works the entire body and is based on the first group of exercises I performed back in 1988! It's a phenomenal workout for the entire body.

The workout is divided into three groups of exercises. Complete each exercise sequentially in group 1, then repeat for a total of three sets before moving on to group 2. Repeat this same approach for groups 2 and 3.

You can scale this workout according to your fitness level by doing one, two, or three sets of each group of exercises.

Group 1	Group 2	Group 3
15 sit-ups or crunches	15 incline push-ups	15 KB upright rows
30 sec of squat jumps	30 sec of star jumps	30 sec of climbers
15 push-ups	15 back extensions	20 calf raises
30 sec of squat jumps	30 sec of star jumps	30 sec of climbers
15 squats	15 RB bent-over rows	15 RB biceps curls
30 sec of plank	30 sec of star jumps	30 sec of climbers
Rest 45–60 sec	Rest 45–60 sec	Rest 45–60 sec
Repeat x 2	*Repeat x 2*	*Repeat x 2*

Cool Down and Stretch

Cool down and stretch protocols ensure that your heart rate lowers and you stretch your body in a manner that helps prevent injury and leads to faster recovery between workouts. These stretches can be undertaken between workouts to aide in faster recovery and reduce muscle soreness.

Refer to AwakenTheSexyWithin.com for your exercise demonstration and cool down and stretching program.

CAUTION: CONSULT A PHYSICIAN BEFORE USING THIS PROGRAM. STOP EXERCISING IF YOU FEEL PAIN, FAINT, DIZZY, OR SHORT OF BREATH.

Workout 2: Tabata Town 1

Warm-up

Your 5-minute warm-up could be as simple as walking around the block, riding a stationary bike, doing 5 minutes of vigorous housework, etc. The important point is to ensure you are appropriately warmed up before performing any of the exercises.

Workout

This is a fantastic workout, allowing you to work at levels of higher intensity for shorter periods of time. The Tabata protocol was invented by a Japanese exercise scientist, Dr. Izumi Tabata. This style of short, intense interval training has been shown to have a dramatic improvement on anaerobic capacity and oxygen uptake.

The aim of this work out is 20 seconds of all-out effort followed by 10 seconds of rest. This is repeated eight times, for a total of 4 minutes. Allow 1–2 minutes of rest between each set. To make this workout more seamless, I suggest you download a free Tabata app for the use of this workout.

For each exercise, perform the eight Tabata rounds before moving on to the next exercise. For example, that means 4 minutes of kettlebell squats (eight rounds of 20 seconds with 10 seconds rest in between). Rest 1–2 minutes, then move to bent-over rows (eight rounds of 20 seconds with 10 seconds rest in between), etc., until all rounds are complete. This can be an intense workout, so pace yourself!

Exercise Description	
Kettlebell squats	Jumping jacks
Bent-over rows	Sit-ups
Push-ups	Upright row
Double crunch	Dips
Shoulder press	Leg raises

Cool Down and Stretch

Cool down and stretch protocols ensure that your heart rate lowers and you stretch your body in a manner that helps prevent injury and leads to faster recovery between workouts. These stretches can be undertaken between workouts to aide in faster recovery and reduce muscle soreness.

Refer to AwakenTheSexyWithin.com for your exercise demonstration and cool down and stretching program.

CAUTION: CONSULT A PHYSICIAN BEFORE USING THIS PROGRAM. STOP EXERCISING IF YOU FEEL PAIN, FAINT, DIZZY, OR SHORT OF BREATH.

Workout 3: Sweat 99 to 1

Warm-up

Your 5-minute warm-up could be as simple as walking around the block, riding a stationary bike, doing 5 minutes of vigorous housework, etc. The important point is to ensure you are appropriately warmed up before performing any of the exercises.

Workout

This is a workout involving a higher than normal volume of repetitions for each exercise, but it's so much fun and an achievement once you complete it. If you are a beginner, you can begin by halving the number of repetitions. If you're intermediate, keep the repetitions as programmed, and make it through the program as far as you can within 60 minutes. If you're advanced, aim to complete the workout as fast as possible. Don't forget to keep a record of your time!

Exercise Description				
Round 1 and 2	**Round 3 and 4**	**Round 5 and 6**	**Round 7 and 8**	**Round 9**
99 mountain climbers	77 alternate leg raise	55 double crunches	33 hip thrusts	11 leg raises
99 bicycle abs	77 side-to-side jumps	55 RB shoulder press	33 KB swings	11 biceps curls
99 squat pulses	77 jumping jacks	55 sumo squats	33 toes tap planks	11 sit-ups
9 push-ups	7 push-ups	5 push-ups	3 push-ups	1 push-up
88 Russian twists	66 butt kicks	44 sit-ups	22 burpees	**End of workout! Congratulations! You made it!**
88 lunges	66 heel touches	44 bent-over rows	22 V sit-ups	
88 high knee	66 squat jumps	44 back extension	22 dips	
8 push-ups	6 push-up	4 push-ups	2 push-ups	

Cool Down and Stretch

Cool down and stretch protocols ensure that your heart rate lowers and you stretch your body in a manner that helps prevent injury and leads to faster recovery between workouts. These stretches can be undertaken between workouts to aide in faster recovery and reduce muscle soreness.

Refer to AwakenTheSexyWithin.com for your exercise demonstration and cool down and stretching program.

CAUTION: CONSULT A PHYSICIAN BEFORE USING THIS PROGRAM. STOP EXERCISING IF YOU FEEL PAIN, FAINT, DIZZY, OR SHORT OF BREATH.

Workout 4: Sexy Legs 1

Warm-up

Your 5-minute warm-up could be as simple as walking around the block, riding a stationary bike, doing 5 minutes of vigorous housework, etc. The important point is to ensure you are appropriately warmed up before performing any of the exercises.

Workout

This is a great workout with only the minimum of equipment required. If you want to do this workout outdoors, find a well-lit area where it is safe to jog, run, or walk without any tripping hazards or causing any disruption to the public. If you would like to do it indoors, then I suggest replacing jogging or running with jogging in place. Each of the exercises is performed for 60 seconds. If you are a beginner, try 30 seconds each round; intermediate, try 45 seconds; and advanced, try 60 seconds.

Round 1 *(10 min)*	Round 2 *(10 min)*	Round 3 *(10 min)*	Round 4 *(10 min)*
1 min of sit-ups	1 min of squat jumps	1 min of power jacks	1 min of leg raises
1 min of squats	1 min of jog or run	1 min of squats	1 min of skip or run
1 min of push-ups	1 min of back extension	1 min of push-ups	1 min of push-ups
1 min of squats	1 min of jog or run	1 min of alt. lunges	1 min of skip or run
1 min of climbers	1 min of leg raises	1 min of squats	1 min of climbers
1 min of squats	1 min of jog or run	1 min of alt. lunges	1 min of skip or run
1 min of dips or sprawl	1 min of plank	1 min of sprawl	1 min of dips or sprawl
1 min of squats	1 min of jog or run	1 min of squats	1 min of skip or run
1 min of sit-ups	1 min of squat jumps	1 min of power jacks	1 min of jackknives
1 min of squats	1 min of jog or run	1 min of squats	1 min of skip or run
1 min rest	1 min rest	1 min rest	1 min rest

Cool Down and Stretch

Cool down and stretch protocols ensure that your heart rate lowers and you stretch your body in a manner that helps prevent injury and leads to faster recovery between workouts. These stretches can be undertaken between workouts to aide in faster recovery and reduce muscle soreness.

Refer to AwakenTheSexyWithin.com for your exercise demonstration and cool down and stretching program.

CAUTION: CONSULT A PHYSICIAN BEFORE USING THIS PROGRAM. STOP EXERCISING IF YOU FEEL PAIN, FAINT, DIZZY, OR SHORT OF BREATH.

Workout 5: The Road to Hell and Back

Warm-up

Your 5-minute warm-up could be as simple as walking around the block, riding a stationary bike, doing 5 minutes of vigorous housework, etc. The important point is to ensure you are appropriately warmed up before performing any of the exercises.

Workout

This is a workout involving a higher than normal volume of repetitions for each exercise, but it's so much fun and an achievement once you complete it. If you are a beginner, you can begin by halving the number of repetitions. If you're intermediate or advanced, keep the repetitions as programmed, and make it through the program as fast as possible. Don't forget to keep a record of your time!

Exercise Description	
1. 100 jumping jacks	9. 60 surrenders
2. 30 jackknives	10. 70 kettlebell swings or climbers
3. 90 lunges	11. 50 leg raises
4. 40 biceps curls	12. 80 double crunches
5. 80 bent-over rows	13. 40 burpees
6. 50 leg raises	14. 90 skipping
7. 70 dips	15. 30 military presses
8. 60 goblet squats	16. 100 heel touches

Cool Down and Stretch

Cool down and stretch protocols ensure that your heart rate lowers and you stretch your body in a manner that helps prevent injury and leads to faster recovery between workouts. These stretches can be undertaken between workouts to aide in faster recovery and reduce muscle soreness.

Refer to AwakenTheSexyWithin.com for your exercise demonstration and cool down and stretching program.

CAUTION: CONSULT A PHYSICIAN BEFORE USING THIS PROGRAM. STOP EXERCISING IF YOU FEEL PAIN, FAINT, DIZZY, OR SHORT OF BREATH.

Workout 6: Pack of Cards 1

Warm-up

Your 5-minute warm-up could be as simple as walking around the block, riding a stationary bike, doing 5 minutes of vigorous housework, etc. The important point is to ensure you are appropriately warmed up before performing any of the exercises.

Workout

This workout is so much fun and involves doing a workout with a pack of playing cards. Each suit of numbered cards (i.e., clubs, diamonds, spades, and hearts) and each face card (i.e., jack, queen, king, and ace) is allocated an exercise, and the number of repetitions will be determined by the number on each card. For example, the eight of hearts requires you to perform 8 burpees.

Prior to commencing, shuffle the deck of cards. When a joker comes up, that's time for a rest—no more than 2 minutes. Set a timer for the length of the workout (20–60 minutes), and complete moving through the deck until your time is up. If you make it through the deck, shuffle and start again. This is a fun workout!

Exercise Description	
Hearts	Burpees
Spades	Push-ups
Clubs	Power jacks
Diamonds	Sit-ups
Ace	20 sec of climbers, 20 sec of jumping jacks, 20 sec of squat jumps, repeat for a total of 2 min. *(30–60-sec rest at the completion of one Ace)*
King	10 double crunches
Queen	10 dips
Jack	10 squats

Cool Down and Stretch

Cool down and stretch protocols ensure that your heart rate lowers and you stretch your body in a manner that helps prevent injury and leads to faster recovery between workouts. These stretches can be undertaken between workouts to aide in faster recovery and reduce muscle soreness.

Refer to AwakenTheSexyWithin.com for your exercise demonstration and cool down and stretching program.

CAUTION: CONSULT A PHYSICIAN BEFORE USING THIS PROGRAM. STOP EXERCISING IF YOU FEEL PAIN, FAINT, DIZZY, OR SHORT OF BREATH.

Workout 7: Partner Smasher 1

Warm-up

Your 5-minute warm-up could be as simple as walking around the block, riding a stationary bike, doing 5 minutes of vigorous housework, etc. The important point is to ensure you are appropriately warmed up before performing any of the exercises.

Workout

This is a great workout that you can perform by yourself, with a buddy, or with multiple buddies! If performing this workout by yourself, set the timer for 60 seconds, work for 45 seconds, and use the remaining 15 seconds to transition to the next exercise. If working with a partner, set the timer to 60 seconds. One person performs one exercise while the other performs the other; swap after each minute, and repeat. If there are multiple buddies, simply team up one or more on each exercise and follow the same sequence.

Round 1	Round 2	Round 3
1. 45 sec of dips ⇔ 45 sec of RB static hold above head	1. Sprawl ⇔ jumping jacks	1. 45 sec of hip thrusts ⇔ 45 sec of hip raises
2. 45 sec of squats ⇔ 45 sec of climbers	2. 45 sec of sit-ups ⇔ 45s sec of plank	2. 45 sec of biceps curls ⇔ 45 sec of triceps extensions
3. 45 sec of push-ups ⇔ 45 sec of suicides	3. Seated row ⇔ jumping jacks	3. 45 sec of double crunches ⇔ 45 sec of back extensions
4. 45 sec of RB shoulder presses ⇔ 45 sec of leg raises	4. 30 sec (each leg) lunges ⇔ 30 sec (each leg) surrenders	4. 45 sec of frog jumps ⇔ 45 sec of bicycle abs
5. 45 sec of plank ⇔ 45 sec of RB upright row static hold	5. Step-ups (1 leg) ⇔ jumping jacks	5. 45 sec of donkey kicks ⇔ 45 sec of heel touches
Rest 45 sec	*Rest 45 sec*	*Rest 45 sec*

Cool Down and Stretch

Cool down and stretch protocols ensure that your heart rate lowers and you stretch your body in a manner that helps prevent injury and leads to faster recovery between workouts. These stretches can be undertaken between workouts to aide in faster recovery and reduce muscle soreness.

Refer to AwakenTheSexyWithin.com for your exercise demonstration and cool down and stretching program.

CAUTION: CONSULT A PHYSICIAN BEFORE USING THIS PROGRAM. STOP EXERCISING IF YOU FEEL PAIN, FAINT, DIZZY, OR SHORT OF BREATH.

Workout 8: Climbing Superset 1

Warm-up

Your 5-minute warm-up could be as simple as walking around the block, riding a stationary bike, doing 5 minutes of vigorous housework, etc. The important point is to ensure you are appropriately warmed up before performing any of the exercises.

Workout

This workout involves supersets of exercises that target each major muscle group. Perform three sets of each exercise, alternating between exercises in each set. You can use dumbbells, kettlebells, or resistance bands for this workout.

If you're outside, find a marker 15 yards away. You will run to this point and back after each exercise until you've completed three sets. If you are indoors, complete 30 seconds of climbers or jumping jacks in between each exercise. At the completion of the three sets, perform the 60 seconds of the allocated high-intensity cardio session.

Station A		Station B	Reps	Cardio (1 min)
Squat and calf raises	⇔	Leg raises	15, 12, 10, or 1 min for each station	Skipping
Surrenders	⇔	Push-ups	15, 12, 10, or 1 min for each station	Squat jumps
Static lunges	⇔	Hip thrusts	15, 12, 10, or 1 min for each station	30-yard sprints or jogging in place
Bent-over rows	⇔	Back extensions	15, 12, 10, or 1 min for each station	Skipping
Double crunches	⇔	Plank	15, 12, 10, or 1 min for each station	Squat jumps
Military presses	⇔	T push-ups	15, 12, 10, or 1 min for each station	30-yard sprints or jogging in place
Russian twists	⇔	Sit-ups	15, 12, 10, or 1 min for each station	Skipping

Cool Down and Stretch

Cool down and stretch protocols ensure that your heart rate lowers and you stretch your body in a manner that helps prevent injury and leads to faster recovery between workouts. These stretches can be undertaken between workouts to aide in faster recovery and reduce muscle soreness.

Refer to AwakenTheSexyWithin.com for your exercise demonstration and cool down and stretching program.

CAUTION: CONSULT A PHYSICIAN BEFORE USING THIS PROGRAM. STOP EXERCISING IF YOU FEEL PAIN, FAINT, DIZZY, OR SHORT OF BREATH.

Workout 9: The Dirty Dozen

Warm-up

Your 5-minute warm-up could be as simple as walking around the block, riding a stationary bike, doing 5 minutes of vigorous housework, etc. The important point is to ensure you are appropriately warmed up before performing any of the exercises.

Workout

The exercises must all be done in order, one after the other. You can take as much rest as required during and between sets; you just need to get the exercises done! Set the timer for between 20 and 60 minutes, and see how far you can get through the workout. If you finish in the designated time, go back to the beginning. Select the number of repetitions you will perform based on your current fitness level: beginner, intermediate, or advanced.

Description	Beginner	Intermediate	Advanced
Squat jumps	30	40	50
Bent-over kettlebell rows	30	40	50
Kettlebell swings	30	40	50
Static lunges with dumbbells or kettlebells	30	40	50
Nose to knee double crunch	30	40	50
Push-ups, whole body to the floor	30	40	50
Back extensions	30	40	50
Thrusts	30	40	50
Kettlebell upright row	30	40	50
Squats with kettlebells	30	40	50
Burpees	30	40	50
Skipping	50	100	150

Cool Down and Stretch

Cool down and stretch protocols ensure that your heart rate lowers and you stretch your body in a manner that helps prevent injury and leads to faster recovery between workouts. These stretches can be undertaken between workouts to aide in faster recovery and reduce muscle soreness.

Refer to AwakenTheSexyWithin.com for your exercise demonstration and cool down and stretching program.

CAUTION: CONSULT A PHYSICIAN BEFORE USING THIS PROGRAM. STOP EXERCISING IF YOU FEEL PAIN, FAINT, DIZZY, OR SHORT OF BREATH.

Workout 10: Four Rounds to Hell 1

Warm-up

Your 5-minute warm-up could be as simple as walking around the block, riding a stationary bike, doing 5 minutes of vigorous housework, etc. The important point is to ensure you are appropriately warmed up before performing any of the exercises.

Workout

This workout involves overloading the muscles, as well as taxing the aerobic system. For beginners, you can vary the number of rounds based on your fitness level. Intermediate and advanced participants should aim to complete the workout in the fastest possible time, adhering to strict form with each exercise.

Round 1	Round 1	Round 3	Round 4
45 sec of lunges	10 squats	10 KB swings	10 bent-over rows
45 sec of side-to-side squats	10 push-ups	10 frog squat jumps	5 RB military press
45 sec of walkdown push-ups	*Repeat for three rounds*	*Repeat for three rounds*	10 sit ups
Repeat for two rounds	30 squats	30 KB swings	
30 sec of plank	30 push-ups	30 frog squat jumps	
30 sec of climbers	*Rest 30 sec*	*Rest 30 sec*	
30 sec of scissor kicks (up)	10 sec of climbers	10 sec of climbers	
30 sec of squat and kick	10 sec of burpees	10 sec of burpees	*Repeat for five rounds*
30 sec of push-ups	10 sec of push-ups	10 sec of push-ups	
30 sec of high knees	10 sec of jumping jacks	10 sec of jumping jacks	
Repeat for two rounds	*Repeat for three rounds*	*Repeat for three rounds*	
Rest 1-min	*Rest 1-min*	*Rest 1-min*	

Cool Down and Stretch

Cool down and stretch protocols ensure that your heart rate lowers and you stretch your body in a manner that helps prevent injury and leads to faster recovery between workouts. These stretches can be undertaken between workouts to aide in faster recovery and reduce muscle soreness.

Refer to AwakenTheSexyWithin.com for your exercise demonstration and cool down and stretching program.

CAUTION: CONSULT A PHYSICIAN BEFORE USING THIS PROGRAM. STOP EXERCISING IF YOU FEEL PAIN, FAINT, DIZZY, OR SHORT OF BREATH.

Workout 11: Killer 90–50, 50–90

Warm-up

Your 5-minute warm-up could be as simple as walking around the block, riding a stationary bike, doing 5 minutes of vigorous housework, etc. The important point is to ensure you are appropriately warmed up before performing any of the exercises.

Workout

This workout has mainly a cardio emphasis. Each round should be for 2–4 minutes, allowing enough time for the pad holder to swap with the boxer and complete approximately 2 minutes of boxing time each.

Round 1	Round 2	Round 3	Round 4
90 push-ups	30 sec of plank	60 sec of high knees	30 sec of plank
10 RB military press	30 sec of leg raises	45 sec of jumping jacks	30 sec of leg raises
80 squat jumps	30 sec of heel touches	30 sec of climbers	30 sec of heel touches
20 RB bent-over rows	*Repeat x 1*	60 sec of skipping	*Repeat x 1*
70 KB swings		60 sec of butt kicks	
30 dips			
60 squats			
40 sit-ups			
50 KB swings			
50 lunges			

Cool Down and Stretch

Cool down and stretch protocols ensure that your heart rate lowers and you stretch your body in a manner that helps prevent injury and leads to faster recovery between workouts. These stretches can be undertaken between workouts to aide in faster recovery and reduce muscle soreness.

Refer to AwakenTheSexyWithin.com for your exercise demonstration and cool down and stretching program.

CAUTION: CONSULT A PHYSICIAN BEFORE USING THIS PROGRAM. STOP EXERCISING IF YOU FEEL PAIN, FAINT, DIZZY, OR SHORT OF BREATH.

Workout 12: Partner Smasher 2

Warm-up

Your 5-minute warm-up could be as simple as walking around the block, riding a stationary bike, doing 5 minutes of vigorous housework, etc. The important point is to ensure you are appropriately warmed up before performing any of the exercises.

Workout

As the name suggests, this workout is great to perform with a buddy but can be performed equally well by yourself. The aim of this workout is to set a marker in place outdoors, at least 30 yards away. While one person walks, jogs, or runs to the marker and back, the partner performs the exercises allocated. Swap turns for two rounds of each exercise. If you are performing this workout by yourself, aim to complete 15 repetitions before completing the walk, jog, or run. Complete two rounds for each exercise. One person does the exercise below for the length of time it takes the partner to run, jog, or walk the designated distance. If you are performing the workout indoors, set a timer for 30 seconds to perform the run, jog, or walk element of the workout and substitute for exercises you can easily perform inside, such as jumping jacks, climbers, high knees, and butt kicks. Use your imagination, and have fun!

Exercise Description		Exercise Description
Dips	⇔	Run, jog, or walk
Squats	⇔	Run, jog, or walk
Push-ups	⇔	Run, jog, or walk
Ball press	⇔	Run, jog, or walk
Plank	⇔	Run, jog, or walk
Sprawl	⇔	Run, jog, or walk
Sit-ups	⇔	Run, jog, or walk
Seated row	⇔	Run, jog, or walk
Lunges	⇔	Run, jog, or walk
Step-ups	⇔	Run, jog, or walk
Triceps extensions	⇔	Run, jog, or walk
Plank with toe taps	⇔	Run, jog, or walk
Double crunches	⇔	Run, jog, or walk
Power jumps	⇔	Run, jog, or walk

Cool Down and Stretch

Cool down and stretch protocols ensure that your heart rate lowers and you stretch your body in a manner that helps prevent injury and leads to faster recovery between workouts. These stretches can be undertaken between workouts to aide in faster recovery and reduce muscle soreness.

Refer to AwakenTheSexyWithin.com for your exercise demonstration and cool down and stretching program.

CAUTION: CONSULT A PHYSICIAN BEFORE USING THIS PROGRAM. STOP EXERCISING IF YOU FEEL PAIN, FAINT, DIZZY, OR SHORT OF BREATH.

Workout 13: Abs and HIIT Smasher 1

Warm-up

Your 5-minute warm-up could be as simple as walking around the block, riding a stationary bike, doing 5 minutes of vigorous housework, etc. The important point is to ensure you are appropriately warmed up before performing any of the exercises.

Workout

This workout is a great one combining abdominal work with Tabata high intense interval training (HIIT). For beginners, you can vary this workout by reducing the abdominal exercises to 30 seconds, and you could cut the number of Tabata sets from eight to four.

Round 1	Round 2	Round 3	Round 4
45 sec of bicycle abs	20 sec of squat jumps ⇔ speed squats (or 10-sec rest), eight sets	45 sec of in and out jumping abs	20 sec of pike push-up x 1, push-up x 1 (10-sec rest) ⇔ jumping jacks, eight sets
45 sec of sky pushes	*Rest 60 sec*	45 sec of side-to-side abs	*Rest 60 sec*
45 sec of punch throughs (left side)	20 sec of burpees ⇔ push-ups (or 10-sec rest), eight sets	45 sec of KB Russian twists	20 sec of hand-to-hand climbers (10-sec rest) ⇔ rocket launchers (10-sec rest), eight sets
45 sec of punch throughs (right side)	*Rest 60 sec*	45 sec of windshield wipers	*Rest 60 sec*
45 sec of accordion crunches	20 sec of fast biceps curls ⇔ climbers (or 10-sec rest), eight sets	45 sec of round the worlds	20 sec of plank walk semicircles (10-sec rest) ⇔ power jacks (10-sec rest), eight sets
60 sec of plank	*Rest 60 sec*	45 sec of Superman leg raises	*Rest 60 sec*
Repeat x 2		*Repeat x 2*	

Cool Down and Stretch

Cool down and stretch protocols ensure that your heart rate lowers and you stretch your body in a manner that helps prevent injury and leads to faster recovery between workouts. These stretches can be undertaken between workouts to aide in faster recovery and reduce muscle soreness.

Refer to AwakenTheSexyWithin.com for your exercise demonstration and cool down and stretching program.

CAUTION: CONSULT A PHYSICIAN BEFORE USING THIS PROGRAM. STOP EXERCISING IF YOU FEEL PAIN, FAINT, DIZZY, OR SHORT OF BREATH.

Workout 14: Total-Body Ab Blaster 1

Warm-up

Your 5-minute warm-up could be as simple as walking around the block, riding a stationary bike, doing 5 minutes of vigorous housework, etc. The important point is to ensure you are appropriately warmed up before performing any of the exercises.

Workout

This is an incredible workout for your whole body, particularly the abdominal muscles. For beginners, you can alter the 60-second rounds to 30 or 45 seconds.

Round 1	Round 2	Round 3	Round 4
60 sec of squat	60 sec of sit-ups	60 sec of incline presses	60 sec of sprawl and punch
30 sec of plank	30 sec of double crunch	30 sec of leg raises	30 sec of Russian twists
60 sec of upright row	60 sec of bent-over row	60 sec of power jumps	60 sec of RB std row
30 sec of plank	30 sec of double crunch	30 sec of leg raises	30 sec of Russian twists
60 sec of push-ups	60 sec of wall squat	60 sec of jackknives	60 sec of lunges
30 sec of plank	30 sec of double crunch	30 sec of leg raises	30 sec of Russian twists
60 sec of power jacks	60 sec of dips	60 sec of back extensions	60 sec of biceps curls
30 sec of plank	30 sec of double crunch	30 sec of leg raises	30 sec of Russian twists
1 min rest and repeat	*1 min rest and repeat*	*1 min rest and repeat*	*1 min rest and repeat*

Cool Down and Stretch

Cool down and stretch protocols ensure that your heart rate lowers and you stretch your body in a manner that helps prevent injury and leads to faster recovery between workouts. These stretches can be undertaken between workouts to aide in faster recovery and reduce muscle soreness.

Refer to AwakenTheSexyWithin.com for your exercise demonstration and cool down and stretching program.

CAUTION: CONSULT A PHYSICIAN BEFORE USING THIS PROGRAM. STOP EXERCISING IF YOU FEEL PAIN, FAINT, DIZZY, OR SHORT OF BREATH.

Workout 15: Max Overload 1

Warm-up

Your 5-minute warm-up could be as simple as walking around the block, riding a stationary bike, doing 5 minutes of vigorous housework, etc. The important point is to ensure you are appropriately warmed up before performing any of the exercises.

Workout

This workout is difficult. It involves a large volume of workload and is not for the fainthearted! It's a great one to do with a buddy or buddies. For beginners, I suggest you halve the number of repetitions for each exercise, and be sure to pace yourself. It is a wonderful achievement to make it to the end of this workout within 60 minutes.

Exercise Description
Set up a cones 30 yards from the starting point. Up and back is one circuit. Complete a total of 15 circuits per person.
500 jab and cross punches (skipping or climbers for those that can't box)
50 burpees (squat jumps or squats for those that can't do burpees, but they must do 2 for every 1 burpee)
150 kettlebell swings
150 double crunches
150 push-ups
150 squats holding a kettlebell
150 climbers
150 side-to-side jumps
150 seated or bent-over rows
150 lunges
150 dips
500 jab and cross punches
Set up a cones 30 yards from the starting point. Up and back is one circuit. Complete a total of 15 circuits per person.

Cool Down and Stretch

Cool down and stretch protocols ensure that your heart rate lowers and you stretch your body in a manner that helps prevent injury and leads to faster recovery between workouts. These stretches can be undertaken between workouts to aide in faster recovery and reduce muscle soreness.

Refer to AwakenTheSexyWithin.com for your exercise demonstration and cool down and stretching program.

CAUTION: CONSULT A PHYSICIAN BEFORE USING THIS PROGRAM. STOP EXERCISING IF YOU FEEL PAIN, FAINT, DIZZY, OR SHORT OF BREATH.

Workout 16: AMRAP Madness 1

Warm-up

Your 5-minute warm-up could be as simple as walking around the block, riding a stationary bike, doing 5 minutes of vigorous housework, etc. The important point is to ensure you are appropriately warmed up before performing any of the exercises.

Workout

AMRAP stands for *as many rounds as possible*, and this workout challenges you to push yourself to your limits. It's a great idea to keep track of how many rounds you're able to complete in the allocated time. Next time you complete the workout, aim to beat the number of rounds. You can alter the length and intensity of this workout by altering the AMRAP time to between 10 and 20 minutes.

20 min AMRAP	1 Round as Fast as Possible	20 min AMRAP	Abdominals
20 squat jumps	21 KB presses	20 Push-ups	15 crunches
15 power jacks	21 bent-over rows	15 double crunches	15 leg raises
10 burpees	15 KB Presses	10 push-ups	60 heel touches
5 power jacks	15 bent-over rows	5 double crunches	30–60 seconds of plank
Rest 1–2 min	9 KB presses	*Rest 1–2 min*	*Repeat x 2*
	9 Bent-over rows		

Cool Down and Stretch

Cool down and stretch protocols ensure that your heart rate lowers and you stretch your body in a manner that helps prevent injury and leads to faster recovery between workouts. These stretches can be undertaken between workouts to aide in faster recovery and reduce muscle soreness.

Refer to AwakenTheSexyWithin.com for your exercise demonstration and cool down and stretching program.

CAUTION: CONSULT A PHYSICIAN BEFORE USING THIS PROGRAM. STOP EXERCISING IF YOU FEEL PAIN, FAINT, DIZZY, OR SHORT OF BREATH.

Workout 17: Six-Packs and Guns

Warm-up
Your 5-minute warm-up could be as simple as walking around the block, riding a stationary bike, doing 5 minutes of vigorous housework, etc. The important point is to ensure you are appropriately warmed up before performing any of the exercises.

Workout
The aim of this workout is to target all areas of the abdominal muscles and the biceps and triceps. For each abdominal exercise, perform for 30–60 seconds, and then move immediately to complete the biceps and triceps exercise for 45–60 seconds. Ideally, you will need a resistance band for this workout.

Exercise Description		Exercise Description
Jackknives	⇔	RB biceps curls
Heel touches	⇔	Dips
Back extensions	⇔	RB hammer curls
Froggy hip-ups	⇔	RB overhead one-arm triceps extensions
Hip drop (right)	⇔	RB biceps curls
Hip drop (left)	⇔	Dips
Stomach flutters	⇔	RB hammer curls
Slow bicycle abs	⇔	RB overhead one-arm triceps extensions
Seated angled V	⇔	RB biceps curls
Plank	⇔	Dips
Snow angels	⇔	RB hammer curls
V-ups	⇔	RB overhead one-arm triceps extensions
Side double leg lift (right)	⇔	RB biceps curls
Side double leg lift (left)	⇔	Dips
Side plank (right)	⇔	RB hammer curls
Side plank (left)	⇔	RB overhead one-arm triceps extensions
Moving spider sprawl	⇔	RB biceps curls
Seated flutter kicks.	⇔	Dips
Hip raises (right)	⇔	RB hammer curls
Hip raises (left)	⇔	RB overhead one-arm triceps extensions
Repeat for a total of three rounds		

Cool Down and Stretch

Cool down and stretch protocols ensure that your heart rate lowers and you stretch your body in a manner that helps prevent injury and leads to faster recovery between workouts. These stretches can be undertaken between workouts to aide in faster recovery and reduce muscle soreness.

Refer to AwakenTheSexyWithin.com for your exercise demonstration and cool down and stretching program.

CAUTION: CONSULT A PHYSICIAN BEFORE USING THIS PROGRAM. STOP EXERCISING IF YOU FEEL PAIN, FAINT, DIZZY, OR SHORT OF BREATH.

Workout 18: 1,000 Reps

Warm-up

Your 5-minute warm-up could be as simple as walking around the block, riding a stationary bike, doing 5 minutes of vigorous housework, etc. The important point is to ensure you are appropriately warmed up before performing any of the exercises.

Workout

The objective of this workout is to complete a total of 1,000 repetitions. The workout contains four sets of 25 repetitions for each of the 10 exercises, done in groups of two exercises at a time in an AB, AB alternating format. For example, do 25 push-ups, then 25 squat jumps, then 25 push-ups, then 25 squat jumps, then move onto exercises 3 and 4. Go all the way through to exercise 10, and then repeat to complete a total of four sets per exercise. For beginners, you can vary the number of repetitions to 10–15 per exercise.

Exercise Description
1. Push-ups
2. Squats
3. Supine plank raises (single leg, alternating)
4. Tuck jumps
5. Burpees
6. Jack knife sit-ups
7. KB swings
8. lunges
9. Bent-over rows
10. Military presses
Repeat for a total of four rounds of 25 reps each, for a total workout of 1,000 repetitions

Cool Down and Stretch

Cool down and stretch protocols ensure that your heart rate lowers and you stretch your body in a manner that helps prevent injury and leads to faster recovery between workouts. These stretches can be undertaken between workouts to aide in faster recovery and reduce muscle soreness.

Refer to AwakenTheSexyWithin.com for your exercise demonstration and cool down and stretching program.

CAUTION: CONSULT A PHYSICIAN BEFORE USING THIS PROGRAM. STOP EXERCISING IF YOU FEEL PAIN, FAINT, DIZZY, OR SHORT OF BREATH.

Workout 19: Sweat It Out—10 to 1

Warm-up

Your 5-minute warm-up could be as simple as walking around the block, riding a stationary bike, doing 5 minutes of vigorous housework, etc. The important point is to ensure you are appropriately warmed up before performing any of the exercises.

Workout

This is a fun workout. Round 1, the 10 exercises need to be completed in order, 10 reps each, followed by a run or alternate exercise. Rounds 2, go down to nine reps per exercise, then eight, etc., until you reach one rep for each exercise.

Exercise Description
1. Bent-over rows
2. Shoulder presses
3. Left leg lunges
4. Right leg lunges
5. Squats
6. Sit-ups
7. Back extension
8. Biceps curls
9. Push-ups
10. Upright rows

Cool Down and Stretch

Cool down and stretch protocols ensure that your heart rate lowers and you stretch your body in a manner that helps prevent injury and leads to faster recovery between workouts. These stretches can be undertaken between workouts to aide in faster recovery and reduce muscle soreness.

Refer to AwakenTheSexyWithin.com for your exercise demonstration and cool down and stretching program.

CAUTION: CONSULT A PHYSICIAN BEFORE USING THIS PROGRAM. STOP EXERCISING IF YOU FEEL PAIN, FAINT, DIZZY, OR SHORT OF BREATH.

Workout 20: Partner Ladder Reps

Warm-up

Your 5-minute warm-up could be as simple as walking around the block, riding a stationary bike, doing 5 minutes of vigorous housework, etc. The important point is to ensure you are appropriately warmed up before performing any of the exercises.

Workout

The aim of this workout is to overload your muscles and test your endurance. Each person needs to partner up with someone, and each pair does alternate repetitions, starting at 1, climbing to 10. While one person exercises, the partner rests. To mix this workout up, start at 10 reps, then move down to 1 rep.

Exercise Description
Sit-ups
Kettlebell sumo squats
Kettlebell upright row
Jumping jacks
Kettlebell clean and press
Kettlebell squats
Burpees
Pushups
Kettlebell bent-over rows
Kettlebell or resistance band biceps curls
Dips

Cool Down and Stretch

Cool down and stretch protocols ensure that your heart rate lowers and you stretch your body in a manner that helps prevent injury and leads to faster recovery between workouts. These stretches can be undertaken between workouts to aide in faster recovery and reduce muscle soreness.

Refer to AwakenTheSexyWithin.com for your exercise demonstration and cool down and stretching program.

CAUTION: CONSULT A PHYSICIAN BEFORE USING THIS PROGRAM. STOP EXERCISING IF YOU FEEL PAIN, FAINT, DIZZY, OR SHORT OF BREATH.

Workout 21: Pyramids and Mountains

Warm-up

Your 5-minute warm-up could be as simple as walking around the block, riding a stationary bike, doing 5 minutes of vigorous housework, etc. The important point is to ensure you are appropriately warmed up before performing any of the exercises.

Workout

This workout is aimed at testing your fitness level. You are competing against yourself or a buddy or two, if they're joining you. The exercises must all be done in order, one after the other. You can take as much rest as required during and between sets; you just need to get the exercises done!

Round 1

	Beginner	Intermediate	Advanced
Run, walk, or jog	200 yards	400 yards	600 yards
10 reps	Crunches	Sit-ups	Sit-ups
20 reps	Squats	KB or sandbag squats	KB or sandbag squats
30 reps	Push-ups	Push-ups	Push-ups
40 reps	Star jumps	Power jacks	Power jacks
50 reps	Squat jumps	Squat jumps	Burpees
40 reps	Star jumps	Power jacks	Power jacks
30 reps	Push-ups	Push-ups	Push-ups
20 reps	Squats	KB or sandbag squats	KB or sandbag squats
10 reps	Crunches	Sit-ups	Sit-ups
Run, walk, or jog	200 yards	400 yards	600 yards

Round 2

Exercise Description
1. 30 sec of sit-ups
2. 30 sec of leg raises
3. 30 sec of heel touches
4. 30–60 sec of plank
Repeat for a total of three rounds

Round 3

Each segment runs for exactly 1 minute. Each person has 60 seconds to perform each of the required 20 exercises. If they finish early, they rest for the remaining time.

Exercise Description	Exercise Description
30 skips + 1 bent-over row	30 skips + 11 bent-over rows
30 skips + 2 bent-over rows	30 skips + 12 bent-over rows
30 skips + 3 bent-over rows	30 skips + 13 bent-over rows
30 skips + 4 bent-over rows	30 skips + 14 bent-over rows
30 skips + 5 bent-over rows	30 skips + 15 bent-over rows
30 skips + 6 bent-over rows	30 skips + 16 bent-over rows
30 skips + 7 bent-over rows	30 skips + 17 bent-over rows
30 skips + 8 bent-over rows	30 skips + 18 bent-over rows
30 skips + 9 bent-over rows	30 skips + 19 bent-over rows
30 skips + 10 bent-over rows	30 skips + 20 bent-over rows

Cool Down and Stretch

Cool down and stretch protocols ensure that your heart rate lowers and you stretch your body in a manner that helps prevent injury and leads to faster recovery between workouts. These stretches can be undertaken between workouts to aide in faster recovery and reduce muscle soreness.

Refer to AwakenTheSexyWithin.com for your exercise demonstration and cool down and stretching program.

CAUTION: CONSULT A PHYSICIAN BEFORE USING THIS PROGRAM. STOP EXERCISING IF YOU FEEL PAIN, FAINT, DIZZY, OR SHORT OF BREATH.

Workout 22: Exploding 50s

Warm-up

Your 5-minute warm-up could be as simple as walking around the block, riding a stationary bike, doing 5 minutes of vigorous housework, etc. The important point is to ensure you are appropriately warmed up before performing any of the exercises.

Workout

As the name describes, 50 reps of one exercise, with a 1-minute rest before you move on to the next exercise. You can vary the intensity of this workout by altering the number of repetitions to 30, 40, or 50.

Exercise Description	
50 squats	50 burpees
50 push-ups	50 leg raises or heel touches
50 tuck jumps	50 dips
50 double crunches	50 mountain climbers
50 KB swings	50 jumping jacks
50 surrenders	50 TRX bent-over rows

Cool Down and Stretch

Cool down and stretch protocols ensure that your heart rate lowers and you stretch your body in a manner that helps prevent injury and leads to faster recovery between workouts. These stretches can be undertaken between workouts to aide in faster recovery and reduce muscle soreness.

Refer to AwakenTheSexyWithin.com for your exercise demonstration and cool down and stretching program.

CAUTION: CONSULT A PHYSICIAN BEFORE USING THIS PROGRAM. STOP EXERCISING IF YOU FEEL PAIN, FAINT, DIZZY, OR SHORT OF BREATH.

Workout 23: Tabata Town 2

Warm-up

Your 5-minute warm-up could be as simple as walking around the block, riding a stationary bike, doing 5 minutes of vigorous housework, etc. The important point is to ensure you are appropriately warmed up before performing any of the exercises.

Workout

This is a fantastic workout, allowing you to work at levels of higher intensity for shorter periods of time. The Tabata protocol was invented by a Japanese exercise scientist, Dr. Izumi Tabata. This style of short, intense interval training has shown to have a dramatic improvement on anaerobic capacity and oxygen uptake.

The aim of this work out is 20 seconds of all-out effort, followed by 10 seconds of rest. This is repeated eight times for a total of 4 minutes. Allow 1–2 minutes rest between each set. To make this workout more seamless, I suggest you download a free Tabata app for the use of this workout.

This is a variation of Tabata town 1. You complete 20 seconds of one exercise, rest for 10 seconds, then move on to the next exercise, for a total of four rounds each.

Exercise Description		Exercise Description
RB military presses	⇔	RB bent-over rows
Dips	⇔	Biceps curls
KB swings	⇔	Jackknives
TRX squats	⇔	Push-ups
Goblet squats	⇔	Plank
One-arm KB rows or RB rows	⇔	Climbers
TRX pistol squats	⇔	Sit-ups
In and out abs	⇔	Heel touches
Squat jumps	⇔	RB overhead hold
Lunges	⇔	RB upright rows

Cool Down and Stretch

Cool down and stretch protocols ensure that your heart rate lowers and you stretch your body in a manner that helps prevent injury and leads to faster recovery between workouts. These stretches can be undertaken between workouts to aide in faster recovery and reduce muscle soreness.

Refer to AwakenTheSexyWithin.com for your exercise demonstration and cool down and stretching program.

CAUTION: CONSULT A PHYSICIAN BEFORE USING THIS PROGRAM. STOP EXERCISING IF YOU FEEL PAIN, FAINT, DIZZY, OR SHORT OF BREATH.

Workout 24: Four Rounds to Hell 2

Warm-up

Your 5-minute warm-up could be as simple as walking around the block, riding a stationary bike, doing 5 minutes of vigorous housework, etc. The important point is to ensure you are appropriately warmed up before performing any of the exercises.

Workout

This is a great workout to complete with a partner, or you can easily do it by yourself.

Round 1	Round 2	Round 3
15 squats	15 burpees	10 push-ups
Wall squat holds	RB military press hold	10 dips
Repeat 3 rounds	*Repeat 3 rounds*	*Repeat 3 rounds*
10 sec of climbers	10 sec of climbers	10 RB step back lunge
10 sec of burpees	10 sec of burpees	10 curtsy squat
10 sec of push-ups	10 sec of push-ups	10 starting step backs
10 sec of jumping jacks	10 sec of jumping jacks	
Repeat for 3 rounds	*Repeat for 3 rounds*	
16 plank and obliques	15 tuck jumps	
Partner static plank	Partner sprawls	
Swap and Repeat 3 rounds	*Swap and Repeat 3 rounds*	*Swap legs and Repeat for 3 rounds*
10 sec of climbers	10 sec of climbers	
10 sec of burpees	10 sec of burpees	
10 sec of push-ups	10 sec of push-ups	
10 sec of jumping jacks	10 sec of jumping jacks	
Repeat for 3 rounds	*Repeat for 3 rounds*	
1 min rest	*1 min rest*	

Cool Down and Stretch

Cool down and stretch protocols ensure that your heart rate lowers and you stretch your body in a manner that helps prevent injury and leads to faster recovery between workouts. These stretches can be undertaken between workouts to aide in faster recovery and reduce muscle soreness.

Refer to AwakenTheSexyWithin.com for your exercise demonstration and cool down and stretching program.

CAUTION: CONSULT A PHYSICIAN BEFORE USING THIS PROGRAM. STOP EXERCISING IF YOU FEEL PAIN, FAINT, DIZZY, OR SHORT OF BREATH.

Workout 25: Total-Body Ab Blaster 2

Warm-up

Your 5-minute warm-up could be as simple as walking around the block, riding a stationary bike, doing 5 minutes of vigorous housework, etc. The important point is to ensure you are appropriately warmed up before performing any of the exercises.

Workout

This is a great workout and is a variation on total-body ab blaster 1. You can vary this workout by altering the time between 30 and 60 seconds to alter the intensity. Make sure you have a timer for this workout.

Round 1	Round 2	Round 3	Round 4
60 sec of squats	60 sec of sit-ups	60 sec of incline push-ups	60 sec of sprawl and punch
30 sec of plank	30 sec of double crunch	30 sec of leg raises	30 sec of Russian twists
60 sec of military presses	60 sec of RB bent-over rows	60 sec of power jumps	60 sec of RB bent-over rows
30 sec of heel touches	30 sec of in and out abs	30 sec of V-ups	30 sec of bicycle abs
60 sec of push-ups	60 sec of wall squats	60 sec of goblet squats	60 sec of lunges
30 sec of plank	30 sec of double crunch	30 sec of leg raises	30 sec of Russian twists
60 sec of split squats	60 sec of dips	60 sec of back extension	60 sec of biceps curls
30 sec of heel touches	30 sec of in and out abs	30 sec of V-ups	30 sec of bicycle abs
1 min rest and repeat	*1 min rest and repeat*	*1 min rest and repeat*	*1 min rest and repeat*

Cool Down and Stretch

Cool down and stretch protocols ensure that your heart rate lowers and you stretch your body in a manner that helps prevent injury and leads to faster recovery between workouts. These stretches can be undertaken between workouts to aide in faster recovery and reduce muscle soreness.

Refer to AwakenTheSexyWithin.com for your exercise demonstration and cool down and stretching program.

CAUTION: CONSULT A PHYSICIAN BEFORE USING THIS PROGRAM. STOP EXERCISING IF YOU FEEL PAIN, FAINT, DIZZY, OR SHORT OF BREATH.

Workout 26: AMRAP Madness 2

Warm-up

Your 5-minute warm-up could be as simple as walking around the block, riding a stationary bike, doing 5 minutes of vigorous housework, etc. The important point is to ensure you are appropriately warmed up before performing any of the exercises.

Workout

AMRAP stands for *as many rounds as possible*, and this workout challenges you to push yourself to your limits. It's a great idea to keep track of how many rounds you're able to complete in the allocated time. Next time you complete the workout, aim to beat the number of rounds. You can alter the length and intensity of this workout by altering the AMRAP time to between 10 and 20 minutes.

Round 1 *20 min of AMRAP*	Round Two	Round Three *20 min of AMRAP*
1. 250 min of run or jog	1. 30 sec of jackknives	1. 60 sec (30 sec each arm)—KB or RB one-arm rows
2. 12 push-ups	2. 30 sec of low plank obliques	2. 30 sec of power jacks (or 20 double crunches)
3. 8 RB military presses	3. 30 sec of in and out abs	3. 30 sec of back extensions
4. 8 bent-over rows	4. 30 sec of knees in knees out	4. 30 sec of climbers or bicycle abs
5. 8 burpees with push-up	5. 30 sec of plank with toe taps	5. 30 sec of KB swings or jumping jacks or bent-over rows
6. 12 butterfly sit-ups	6. 30 sec of heel touches	6. 30 sec of deep squats with 2 pulses (or 30 push-ups)
	7. 30 sec of sit-ups with 10 punches	7. 30 sec of dips or RB triceps extensions
	8. 30 sec of sprawl with power punches	8. 60 sec of run or jog
Rest 1–2 min	9. 30 sec of reverse crunch	
	10. 30 sec of double crunch	

Cool Down and Stretch

Cool down and stretch protocols ensure that your heart rate lowers and you stretch your body in a manner that helps prevent injury and leads to faster recovery between workouts. These stretches can be undertaken between workouts to aide in faster recovery and reduce muscle soreness.

Refer to AwakenTheSexyWithin.com for your exercise demonstration and cool down and stretching program.

CAUTION: CONSULT A PHYSICIAN BEFORE USING THIS PROGRAM. STOP EXERCISING IF YOU FEEL PAIN, FAINT, DIZZY, OR SHORT OF BREATH.

Workout 27: OMG No More Squats Please!

Warm-up

Your 5-minute warm-up could be as simple as walking around the block, riding a stationary bike, doing 5 minutes of vigorous housework, etc. The important point is to ensure you are appropriately warmed up before performing any of the exercises.

Workout

This is a great workout with only the minimum of equipment required. You need to find some steps or park benches or a solid chair to assist with the workout.

Each of the exercises is performed to time with a total of five rounds being completed. This workout should take about 50 minutes.

Round 1	Round 2	Round 3	Round 4
1 min of step-ups	1 min of log jump-overs	1 min of log power jacks	1 min of step-ups
1 min of stairs	1 min of jog or run	1 min of stairs	1 min of skip or run
1 min of log push-ups	1 min of RB rows	1 min of log push-ups	1 min of log push-ups
1 min of stairs	1 min of jog or run	1 min of stairs	1 min of skip or run
1 min of log climbers	1 min of step-ups	1 min of squats	1 min of log climbers
1 min of stairs	1 min of jog or run	1 min of stairs	1 min of skip or run
1 min of dips	1 min of RB biceps curls	1 min of log sprawl	1 min of dips
1 min of stairs	1 min of jog or run	1 min of stairs	1 min of skip or run
1 min of step-ups	1 min of log jump-overs	1 min of log power jacks	1 min of step-ups
1 min of stairs	1 min of jog or run	1 min of stairs	1 min of skip or run
1 min rest	*1 min rest*	*1 min rest*	*1 min rest*

Cool Down and Stretch

Cool down and stretch protocols ensure that your heart rate lowers and you stretch your body in a manner that helps prevent injury and leads to faster recovery between workouts. These stretches can be undertaken between workouts to aide in faster recovery and reduce muscle soreness.

Refer to AwakenTheSexyWithin.com for your exercise demonstration and cool down and stretching program.

CAUTION: CONSULT A PHYSICIAN BEFORE USING THIS PROGRAM. STOP EXERCISING IF YOU FEEL PAIN, FAINT, DIZZY, OR SHORT OF BREATH.

Workout 28: Pack of Cards 2

Warm-up

Your 5-minute warm-up could be as simple as walking around the block, riding a stationary bike, doing 5 minutes of vigorous housework, etc. The important point is to ensure you are appropriately warmed up before performing any of the exercises.

Workout

This workout involves doing a workout with a pack of normal playing cards. Each suit of card is allocated an exercise, and you perform the number of repetitions on the card.

Shuffle the deck of cards before you start. When a joker comes up, that's time to have a rest for up to 2 minutes. This is a fun workout and hard!

Description	
Card	**Exercise**
Hearts	Lunges
Spades	Frog jumps or squat and hold
Clubs	Plank
Diamonds	Double crunch
Aces =	10 sec each of burpees, push-ups, climbers, jumping jacks. Complete for a total of four rounds = 2 min *(30–60 sec rest at the completion of one ace)*
Kings	10 sitting abdominal knees in and out crunch
Queen	10 burpees
Jack	10 jackknives

Cool Down and Stretch

Cool down and stretch protocols ensure that your heart rate lowers and you stretch your body in a manner that helps prevent injury and leads to faster recovery between workouts. These stretches can be undertaken between workouts to aide in faster recovery and reduce muscle soreness.

Refer to AwakenTheSexyWithin.com for your exercise demonstration and cool down and stretching program.

CAUTION: CONSULT A PHYSICIAN BEFORE USING THIS PROGRAM. STOP EXERCISING IF YOU FEEL PAIN, FAINT, DIZZY, OR SHORT OF BREATH.

Workout 29: Climbing Superset 2

Warm-up

Your 5-minute warm-up could be as simple as walking around the block, riding a stationary bike, doing 5 minutes of vigorous housework, etc. The important point is to ensure you are appropriately warmed up before performing any of the exercises.

Workout

This workout involves supersets of exercises that target each major muscle group. Perform three sets of each exercise, alternating between exercises in each set. You can use dumbbells, kettlebells, or resistance bands for this workout.

If you're outside, find a marker 15 yards away. You will run to this point and back after each exercise until you've completed three sets. If you are indoors, complete 30 seconds of climbers or jumping jacks in between each exercise. At the completion of the three sets, perform the 60 seconds of the allocated high-intensity cardio session.

Station A (RBs)		Station B (Mats)	Reps	60 Sec of High-Intensity Cardio
Military presses	⇔	Leg raises	15, 12, 10, or 1 min for each station	10 sec climbers, burpees, push-ups, jumping jacks
KB swings	⇔	Push-ups	15, 12, 10, or 1 min for each station	Skipping
KB deadlifts	⇔	Plank and lateral drag	15, 12, 10, or 1 min for each station	Virtual boxing, jab and cross
Squats and lunges	⇔	Double crunches	15, 12, 10, or 1 min for each station	10 sec climbers, burpees, push-ups, jumping jacks
RB bent-over rows	⇔	Plank and knees to opposite shoulder	15, 12, 10, or 1 min for each station	Skipping
KB upright rows	⇔	Squat jumps	15, 12, 10, or 1 min for each station	Virtual boxing, jab and cross
KB, bag, or ball Russian twists	⇔	Calf raises	15, 12, 10, or 1 min for each station	

Cool Down and Stretch

Cool down and stretch protocols ensure that your heart rate lowers and you stretch your body in a manner that helps prevent injury and leads to faster recovery between workouts. These stretches can be undertaken between workouts to aide in faster recovery and reduce muscle soreness.

Refer to AwakenTheSexyWithin.com for your exercise demonstration and cool down and stretching program.

CAUTION: CONSULT A PHYSICIAN BEFORE USING THIS PROGRAM. STOP EXERCISING IF YOU FEEL PAIN, FAINT, DIZZY, OR SHORT OF BREATH.

Workout 30: Leg Smasher

Warm-up

Your 5-minute warm-up could be as simple as walking around the block, riding a stationary bike, doing 5 minutes of vigorous housework, etc. The important point is to ensure you are appropriately warmed up before performing any of the exercises.

Workout

The aim of this workout is to completely fatigue the legs. This is a tough workout!

Exercise Description	
12 KB squats	20 calf raises
10 alternating lunges each side	15 hip thrusts
12 sumo KB sumo squats	15 hip raises each side
10 alternating side lunges each side	10 KB one-legged deadlifts each side
30 side-to-side jumps	20 step-ups
25 power jacks	16 surrenders
35 star jumps	
1 min rest, repeat x 2	

Cool Down and Stretch

Cool down and stretch protocols ensure that your heart rate lowers and you stretch your body in a manner that helps prevent injury and leads to faster recovery between workouts. These stretches can be undertaken between workouts to aide in faster recovery and reduce muscle soreness.

Refer to AwakenTheSexyWithin.com for your exercise demonstration and cool down and stretching program.

CAUTION: CONSULT A PHYSICIAN BEFORE USING THIS PROGRAM. STOP EXERCISING IF YOU FEEL PAIN, FAINT, DIZZY, OR SHORT OF BREATH.

Workout 31: Circuit Intensity 1

Warm-up

Your 5-minute warm-up could be as simple as walking around the block, riding a stationary bike, doing 5 minutes of vigorous housework, etc. The important point is to ensure you are appropriately warmed up before performing any of the exercises.

Workout

This workout involves a fun circuit, based on timed intervals for each set. You can set one, two, three, or more people per exercise and rotate at the end of each time slot. This is quite an intense workout, with no rest until all the exercises in each round are completed. You could do this workout to time or to number of reps, depending on the size of the group.

Round 1	Round 2	Round 3	Round 4
30 sec of heel touches	45 sec of burpees	45 sec of squat globe jumps	60 sec of sprawl and punch
30 sec of plank	45 sec lunges	45 sec bear crawl	30 sec of star jumps
30 sec of double crunches	45 sec step-ups	45 sec log jump overs	60 sec of resistance band (RB) bent-over rows
30 sec of plank with knee to opposite shoulder	45 sec of frog jumps	45 sec side-to-side ski jumps	30 sec of plank toe taps
30 sec of plank with toe tap	45 sec of push-ups with ball	45 sec of squat jumps	60 sec of step-ups
30 sec of windshield wipers	45 sec of step-ups	45 sec of side-to-side ski jumps	30 sec of Russian twists
30 sec of heel touches	45 sec of lunges	45 sec of log jump overs	60 sec of triceps extensions
30 sec of plank	45 sec of burpees	45 sec of bear crawl	30 sec of V-ups
30 sec of double crunches	45 sec of plank	45 sec of squat globe jumps	60 sec of back extensions
1 min rest and repeat	*1 min rest*	*1 min rest*	*1 min rest and repeat*

Cool Down and Stretch

Cool down and stretch protocols ensure that your heart rate lowers and you stretch your body in a manner that helps prevent injury and leads to faster recovery between workouts. These stretches can be undertaken between workouts to aide in faster recovery and reduce muscle soreness.

Refer to AwakenTheSexyWithin.com for your exercise demonstration and cool down and stretching program.

CAUTION: CONSULT A PHYSICIAN BEFORE USING THIS PROGRAM. STOP EXERCISING IF YOU FEEL PAIN, FAINT, DIZZY, OR SHORT OF BREATH.

Workout 32: Tabata Town 3

Warm-up

Your 5-minute warm-up could be as simple as walking around the block, riding a stationary bike, doing 5 minutes of vigorous housework, etc. The important point is to ensure you are appropriately warmed up before performing any of the exercises.

Workout

This is a fantastic workout, allowing you to work at levels of higher intensity for shorter periods of time. The Tabata protocol was invented by a Japanese exercise scientist, Dr. Izumi Tabata.

This is a variation of Tabata town 1 and 2. For exercise 1, you complete 20 seconds of one exercise, rest for 10 seconds, then move on to the next exercise, for a total of four rounds each. For exercise 2, you complete the entire eight Tabata rounds on the one exercise, and so on through the workout, where exercise 3 follows the same format as exercise 1.

Exercise Description		Exercise Description
Sit up	⇔	Leg raises
Squat pulses	⇔	Squat pulses
Push-ups	⇔	Plank
Jumping jacks	⇔	Jumping jacks
Upright row	⇔	biceps curls
Dips	⇔	Climbers
Squat jumps	⇔	Wall squat
Heel touches	⇔	Double crunch
Bicycle abs	⇔	Bicycle abs
Burpees	⇔	Sprawl

Cool Down and Stretch

Cool down and stretch protocols ensure that your heart rate lowers and you stretch your body in a manner that helps prevent injury and leads to faster recovery between workouts. These stretches can be undertaken between workouts to aide in faster recovery and reduce muscle soreness.

Refer to AwakenTheSexyWithin.com for your exercise demonstration and cool down and stretching program.

CAUTION: CONSULT A PHYSICIAN BEFORE USING THIS PROGRAM. STOP EXERCISING IF YOU FEEL PAIN, FAINT, DIZZY, OR SHORT OF BREATH.

Workout 33: The 48s

Warm-up

Your 5-minute warm-up could be as simple as walking around the block, riding a stationary bike, doing 5 minutes of vigorous housework, etc. The important point is to ensure you are appropriately warmed up before performing any of the exercises.

Workout

If you love variety, this workout is for you. A total of 48 different exercises are included in this workout. Each exercise is prescribed for 60 seconds, but you can alter the intensity by varying the time to 30–60 seconds.

Round 1 (1 min each)	Round 2 (1 min each)	Round 3 (1 min each)	Round 4 (1 min each)
Heel touches	Plank toe taps	V sit-ups	KB swings
Push-ups	RB biceps curls	Jumping jacks	Frog jumps
Plank	Double crunch	Jackknives	KB side bends
Lunges	Burpees	RB flies	RB chest press
Climbers	Sit-ups	Left side plank	Flutter kicks
Dips	Sprawl	Back extensions	Squat jumps
Reverse crunch	In and out abs	Right side plank	Butterfly sit-ups
Squat	Skipping	Hip thrusts	RB bent-over row
Bicycle abs	Side-to-side abs	Sit up and 10 punches	Sumo squats
RB military press	RB upright row	RB hammer curls	Sprawl and punch
Leg raises	Plank and knees	Side-to-side jumps	Russian twists
Wall squat	Alt. leg raises	RB triceps extension	Windshield wipers
1 min rest	*1 min rest*	*1 min rest*	*1 min rest*

Cool Down and Stretch

Cool down and stretch protocols ensure that your heart rate lowers and you stretch your body in a manner that helps prevent injury and leads to faster recovery between workouts. These stretches can be undertaken between workouts to aide in faster recovery and reduce muscle soreness.

Refer to AwakenTheSexyWithin.com for your exercise demonstration and cool down and stretching program.

CAUTION: CONSULT A PHYSICIAN BEFORE USING THIS PROGRAM. STOP EXERCISING IF YOU FEEL PAIN, FAINT, DIZZY, OR SHORT OF BREATH.

Workout 34: Boxing Body Tone 1

Warm-up

Your 5-minute warm-up could be as simple as walking around the block, riding a stationary bike, doing 5 minutes of vigorous housework, etc. The important point is to ensure you are appropriately warmed up before performing any of the exercises.

Workout

This is a great workout to do with a buddy but can easily be performed by yourself. The boxing can be simulated with virtual boxing, performing air jab and cross punches. You can vary the intensity of this workout by reducing the time of each exercise to 30–60 seconds.

Round 1	Round 2	Round 3	Round 4
1 min (partner) sit-ups and 10 punches	45 sec of squat, normal	1 min (partner) sit-ups and 10 punches	45 sec of squat, normal
1 min (partner) RB military press or jab and cross	45 sec of static lunges	1 min (partner) RB military press or jab and cross	45 sec of static lunges
1 min (partner) leg raise	45 sec of squat, sumo	1 min (partner) leg raise and throw	45 sec of squat, sumo
Repeat twice then swap over and repeat	45 sec of thrusts	*Repeat twice then swap over and repeat*	45 sec of thrusts
	45 sec of hip thrusts		45 sec of hip thrusts
	45 sec of wall hold squat		45 sec of wall hold squat
	45 sec of squat jumps		45 sec of squat jumps

Round 5	Round 6	Round 7
45 sec of push-ups	1 min (partner) sit-ups and 10 punches	45 sec of push-ups
45 sec of plank	1 min (partner) RB military press or jab and cross	45 sec of plank
45 sec of dips	1 min (partner) leg raise and throw	45 sec of dips
45 sec of upright rows	*Repeat twice then swap over and repeat*	45 sec of upright rows
45 sec of biceps curls		45 sec of biceps curls
45 sec of plank		45 sec of plank
45 sec of shoulder press		45 sec of RB military press

Cool Down and Stretch

Cool down and stretch protocols ensure that your heart rate lowers and you stretch your body in a manner that helps prevent injury and leads to faster recovery between workouts. These stretches can be undertaken between workouts to aide in faster recovery and reduce muscle soreness.

Refer to AwakenTheSexyWithin.com for your exercise demonstration and cool down and stretching program.

CAUTION: CONSULT A PHYSICIAN BEFORE USING THIS PROGRAM. STOP EXERCISING IF YOU FEEL PAIN, FAINT, DIZZY, OR SHORT OF BREATH.

Workout 35: Quads on Fire

Warm-up

Your 5-minute warm-up could be as simple as walking around the block, riding a stationary bike, doing 5 minutes of vigorous housework, etc. The important point is to ensure you are appropriately warmed up before performing any of the exercises.

Workout

This is an intense workout, taxing mainly your aerobic capacity. You will need access to a set of stairs, a bench, or a solid chair to complete the stair and step-up portion of the workout. You can vary the intensity of this workout by altering the time between 30 and 60 seconds.

Round 1	Round 2	Round 3	Round 4	Round 5
30 sec of heel touches	20 sec of jumping jacks	60 sec of step-ups	60 sec of log power jacks	60 sec of 10 punches ⇔ 3 push-ups
30 sec of plank	60 sec of squat jumps	60 sec of stairs	60 sec of stairs	60 sec of 4 knees ⇔ 4 squat jumps
30 sec of double crunches	30 sec of sumo squats	60 sec of log push-ups	60 sec of log push-ups	60 sec of 10 punches ⇔ 4 knees ⇔ 4 squat jumps
30 sec of plank with knee to opposite shoulder	30 sec of high knees	60 sec of stairs	60 sec of stairs	*Swap and repeat*
30 sec of plank with toe tap	10 sec of squat jumps	60 sec of log climbers	60 sec of squats	20 sec of jab and cross ⇔ 20 sec of burpees ⇔ 20 sec of jab and cross
30 sec of windshield wipers	20 sec of sumo squats	60 sec of stairs	60 sec of stairs	Upper cut—20 sec ⇔ Sprawl—20 sec ⇔ Upper cuts—20 sec
30 sec of heel touches	30 sec of butt kicks	60 sec of dips	60 sec of log sprawl	Blocks—20 sec ⇔ Push-ups—20 sec ⇔ Blocks—20 sec
30 sec of plank	10 sec of squat jumps	60 sec of stairs	60 sec of stairs	*Swap and Repeat*
30 sec of double crunches	30 sec of sumo squats	60 sec of step-ups	60 sec of log power jacks	
30 sec of plank with knee to opposite shoulder	20 sec of jumping jacks	60 sec of stairs	60 sec of stairs	
1 min rest	*1 min rest and repeat*	*1 min rest*	*1 min rest*	*1 min rest*

Cool Down and Stretch

Cool down and stretch protocols ensure that your heart rate lowers and you stretch your body in a manner that helps prevent injury and leads to faster recovery between workouts. These stretches can be undertaken between workouts to aide in faster recovery and reduce muscle soreness.

Refer to AwakenTheSexyWithin.com for your exercise demonstration and cool down and stretching program.

CAUTION: CONSULT A PHYSICIAN BEFORE USING THIS PROGRAM. STOP EXERCISING IF YOU FEEL PAIN, FAINT, DIZZY, OR SHORT OF BREATH.

Workout 36: Exhaustion Workout 1

Warm-up

Your 5-minute warm-up could be as simple as walking around the block, riding a stationary bike, doing 5 minutes of vigorous housework, etc. The important point is to ensure you are appropriately warmed up before performing any of the exercises.

Workout

This is great workout based on timed intervals. You can vary the intensity by altering the timed segments of the workout.

Round 1 *Complete all the exercises below within 2 min*	Round 2 *45 sec on each station 15 sec rest in between*	Round 3 *45 sec on each station 15 sec rest in between*
12 push-ups	Push-ups	Sit up with 10 punches
15 squats	Squats	Burpees
80 punches	Punches	Leg raises
20 jumping jacks	Jumping jacks	
15 squat jumps	Squat jumps	*1 min rest*
Rest 1 min and repeat x 2	*1 min rest*	
Round 4	**Round 5**	**Round 6**
1 min of wall squat and hold	45 sec dips	30 sec burpees
30 sec of power jacks	45 sec squats	30 sec squats with 2 pulses
30 sec of sprawls	45 sec push-ups	
1 min of lunges		
Rest 1 min and repeat	*Rest 1 min and repeat*	*Repeat. x 3*

Cool Down and Stretch

Cool down and stretch protocols ensure that your heart rate lowers and you stretch your body in a manner that helps prevent injury and leads to faster recovery between workouts. These stretches can be undertaken between workouts to aide in faster recovery and reduce muscle soreness.

Refer to AwakenTheSexyWithin.com for your exercise demonstration and cool down and stretching program.

CAUTION: CONSULT A PHYSICIAN BEFORE USING THIS PROGRAM. STOP EXERCISING IF YOU FEEL PAIN, FAINT, DIZZY, OR SHORT OF BREATH.

Workout 37: Buns of Steel

Warm-up

Your 5-minute warm-up could be as simple as walking around the block, riding a stationary bike, doing 5 minutes of vigorous housework, etc. The important point is to ensure you are appropriately warmed up before performing any of the exercises.

Workout

The aim of this workout is to target the legs and abdominal muscles—specifically, the glutes (butt), quadriceps (front of the leg), and hamstrings (back of the leg); upper, lower, and side abdominal muscles; as well as the core. Complete the entire program through, then repeat up to three times in the time allotted. You can vary the intensity of this workout by altering the time to between 30 and 60 seconds.

Exercise Description *60 sec each exercise*		Exercise Description *30 sec each exercise*
Squat	⇔	Jackknives
Forward lunges	⇔	Plank
KB Thrusts	⇔	Leg raises (2 legs)
KB stiff leg deadlift	⇔	KB Russian twists
Glute bridge or Hip thrusts	⇔	Jackknives
TRX Pistol squats	⇔	Double crunches
KB swings	⇔	Plank
Side lunges	⇔	Reverse crunch
Lying hip abductors	⇔	Bicycle abs
Good mornings	⇔	KB Russian twists
Calf raises	⇔	Sit-ups
Repeat for a total of three rounds		

Cool Down and Stretch

Cool down and stretch protocols ensure that your heart rate lowers and you stretch your body in a manner that helps prevent injury and leads to faster recovery between workouts. These stretches can be undertaken between workouts to aide in faster recovery and reduce muscle soreness.

Refer to AwakenTheSexyWithin.com for your exercise demonstration and cool down and stretching program.

CAUTION: CONSULT A PHYSICIAN BEFORE USING THIS PROGRAM. STOP EXERCISING IF YOU FEEL PAIN, FAINT, DIZZY, OR SHORT OF BREATH.

Workout 38: AMRAP Madness 3

Warm-up

Your 5-minute warm-up could be as simple as walking around the block, riding a stationary bike, doing 5 minutes of vigorous housework, etc. The important point is to ensure you are appropriately warmed up before performing any of the exercises.

Workout

This is a great workout to test your endurance. Set your timer to between 1 and 3 minutes, and aim to complete as many repetitions as you can within the designated time. You need to keep count of the number of repetitions you complete. Record them and keep the details somewhere you can compare to the next time you complete this workout.

Exercise Description
1. Dips
2. Squats
3. Push-ups
4. RB military presses
5. Burpees
6. Partner hand slaps
7. Sit-ups
8. Seated row
9. Dumbbell punches
10. Side-to-side jumps
11. Sprawl with alternate toe taps
12. RB or dumbbell front raises
13. RB or dumbbell lateral raises

Cool Down and Stretch

Cool down and stretch protocols ensure that your heart rate lowers and you stretch your body in a manner that helps prevent injury and leads to faster recovery between workouts. These stretches can be undertaken between workouts to aide in faster recovery and reduce muscle soreness.

Refer to AwakenTheSexyWithin.com for your exercise demonstration and cool down and stretching program.

CAUTION: CONSULT A PHYSICIAN BEFORE USING THIS PROGRAM. STOP EXERCISING IF YOU FEEL PAIN, FAINT, DIZZY, OR SHORT OF BREATH.

Workout 39: Climbing Superset 3

Warm-up

Your 5-minute warm-up could be as simple as walking around the block, riding a stationary bike, doing 5 minutes of vigorous housework, etc. The important point is to ensure you are appropriately warmed up before performing any of the exercises.

Workout

This workout involves supersets of exercises that target each major muscle group. Perform 3 sets of each exercise, alternating between exercises in each set. You can use dumbbells, kettlebells, or resistance bands for this workout.

If you're outside, find a marker 15 yards away. You will run to this point and back after each exercise until you've completed three sets. If you are indoors, complete 30 seconds of climbers or jumping jacks in between each exercise. At the completion of the three sets, perform the 60 seconds of the allocated high-intensity cardio session.

Station A		Station B	Reps	60 sec Cardio
Ball or sand bag slams	⇔	Leg raises	15, 12, 10, or 1 min for each station	10 sec climbers, burpees, push-ups, jumping jacks
KB swings	⇔	Push-ups	15, 12, 10, or 1 min for each station	Frog jumps
Lunges	⇔	Plank and lateral drag	15, 12, 10, or 1 min for each station	Squat jumps
Ball or sand bag drop and turns	⇔	Double crunches	15, 12, 10, or 1 min for each station	10 sec climbers, burpees, push-ups, jumping jacks
Ball or sand bag throws	⇔	Plank and knees to opposite shoulder	15, 12, 10, or 1 min for each station	Frog Jumps
RB upright rows	⇔	Squats	15, 12, 10, or 1 min for each station	Squat jumps
KB, bag, or ball Russian twists	⇔	Sit-ups	15, 12, 10, or 1 min for each station	**Rest**

Cool Down and Stretch

Cool down and stretch protocols ensure that your heart rate lowers and you stretch your body in a manner that helps prevent injury and leads to faster recovery between workouts. These stretches can be undertaken between workouts to aide in faster recovery and reduce muscle soreness.

Refer to AwakenTheSexyWithin.com for your exercise demonstration and cool down and stretching program.

CAUTION: CONSULT A PHYSICIAN BEFORE USING THIS PROGRAM. STOP EXERCISING IF YOU FEEL PAIN, FAINT, DIZZY, OR SHORT OF BREATH.

Workout 40: Tabata Town 4

Warm-up

Your 5-minute warm-up could be as simple as walking around the block, riding a stationary bike, doing 5 minutes of vigorous housework, etc. The important point is to ensure you are appropriately warmed up before performing any of the exercises.

Workout

This is a fantastic workout, allowing you to work at levels of higher intensity for shorter periods of time. The Tabata protocol was invented by a Japanese exercise scientist, Dr. Izumi Tabata. The aim of this work out is 20 seconds of all-out effort, followed by 10 seconds of rest. This is repeated eight times for a total of 4 minutes. Allow 1–2 minutes of rest between each set. To make this workout more seamless, I suggest you download a free Tabata app for the use of this workout. For each exercise, perform the eight Tabata rounds before moving on to the next exercise. This can be an intense workout, so pace yourself!

Exercise Description
1. Sit-ups
2. Push-ups
3. Back extensions
4. Split squats
5. RB military presses
6. RB bent-over rows
7. Hip thrusts
8. RB upright rows
9. Dips
10. RB biceps curls
11. Pistol squats
12. Lunges
13. Side-to-side lunges
14. Leg raises
15. Calf raises

Cool Down and Stretch

Cool down and stretch protocols ensure that your heart rate lowers and you stretch your body in a manner that helps prevent injury and leads to faster recovery between workouts. These stretches can be undertaken between workouts to aide in faster recovery and reduce muscle soreness.

Refer to AwakenTheSexyWithin.com for your exercise demonstration and cool down and stretching program.

CAUTION: CONSULT A PHYSICIAN BEFORE USING THIS PROGRAM. STOP EXERCISING IF YOU FEEL PAIN, FAINT, DIZZY, OR SHORT OF BREATH.

Workout 41: Total-Body Ab Blaster 3

Warm-up
Your 5-minute warm-up could be as simple as walking around the block, riding a stationary bike, doing 5 minutes of vigorous housework, etc. The important point is to ensure you are appropriately warmed up before performing any of the exercises.

Workout
This is a great workout, with plenty of variety. Note that round 1 involves setting a timer for 14 minutes and completing AMRAP (as many rounds as possible) within that time. Rounds 2–4 are based on 30- and 60-second rounds. You can vary the intensity of the workout by altering the timed intervals.

Round 1 AMRAP 14 min	Round 2	Round 3	Round 4
70 skips	60 sec of shoulder press	60 sec of wall push-ups	60 sec of sprawl and punch
7 burpees	30 sec of double crunch	30 sec of leg raises	30 sec of star jumps
7 push-ups	60 sec of upright row	60 sec of squat jumps	60 sec of RB std row
7 squats	30 sec of plank	30 sec of knees in and out	30 sec of plank toe taps
7 bent-over rows	60 sec of wall squat hold	60 sec of lunges	60 sec of step-ups
7 sit-ups	30 sec of heel touches	30 sec of plank obliques	30 sec of Russian twists
7 power jack	60 sec of dips	60 sec of back extension	60 sec of RB triceps extensions
7 sprints (20–30 min)	60 sec of climbers	30 sec of jackknives	30 sec of V-ups
1 min rest	*1 min rest and repeat*	*1 min rest and repeat*	*1 min rest and repeat*

Cool Down and Stretch

Cool down and stretch protocols ensure that your heart rate lowers and you stretch your body in a manner that helps prevent injury and leads to faster recovery between workouts. These stretches can be undertaken between workouts to aide in faster recovery and reduce muscle soreness.

Refer to AwakenTheSexyWithin.com for your exercise demonstration and cool down and stretching program.

CAUTION: CONSULT A PHYSICIAN BEFORE USING THIS PROGRAM. STOP EXERCISING IF YOU FEEL PAIN, FAINT, DIZZY, OR SHORT OF BREATH.

Workout 42: Jumping 40s

Warm-up

Your 5-minute warm-up could be as simple as walking around the block, riding a stationary bike, doing 5 minutes of vigorous housework, etc. The important point is to ensure you are appropriately warmed up before performing any of the exercises.

Workout

Set up four stations (or more, depending on number of participants) and have one or more people begin at each station. Rotate after each set is performed.

Round 1	Round 2	Round 3
10 push-ups	30 sec of crunches	10 RB bent-over rows
40 jumping jacks	30 sec of leg raises	40 jumping jacks
10 dips	30 sec of leg raise criss-crosses	10 good mornings
40 jumping jacks	30 sec of plank	40 jumping jacks
10 squats	30 sec of bicycle abs	10 back extensions
40 jumping jacks	30 sec of heel touches	40 jumping jacks
10 burpees	30 sec of back extensions	10 climbers
40 jumping jacks	30 sec of plank	40 jumping jacks
Repeat two or three times	*Repeat*	*Repeat two or three times*

Cool Down and Stretch

Cool down and stretch protocols ensure that your heart rate lowers and you stretch your body in a manner that helps prevent injury and leads to faster recovery between workouts. These stretches can be undertaken between workouts to aide in faster recovery and reduce muscle soreness.

Refer to AwakenTheSexyWithin.com for your exercise demonstration and cool down and stretching program.

CAUTION: CONSULT A PHYSICIAN BEFORE USING THIS PROGRAM. STOP EXERCISING IF YOU FEEL PAIN, FAINT, DIZZY, OR SHORT OF BREATH.

Workout 43: Beach Legs

Warm-up

Your 5-minute warm-up could be as simple as walking around the block, riding a stationary bike, doing 5 minutes of vigorous housework, etc. The important point is to ensure you are appropriately warmed up before performing any of the exercises.

Workout

This workout is a great one to get you beach ready and toning those sexy legs of yours! You can vary the intensity of this workout by varying the timed intervals.

Round 1	Round 2
1. 45 sec of good mornings	1. 60 sec of sit-ups
2. 60 sec of lunges	2. 45 sec of hip thrusts, alternating sides
3. 30 sec of side-to-side jumps	3. 30 sec of butt kicks to roof, alternate sides
4. 45 sec of plank	4. 30 sec of climbers
5. 30 sec of bent-over rows, swap and repeat	5. 60 sec of lunges
6. 45 sec of squats	6. 45 sec of bent-over rows
7. 30 sec of running in place with high knees	7. 30 sec of alternating side plank
8. 45 sec of wall squat	8. 60 sec of plank
9. 30 sec of double crunches	*Repeat two or three times*
10. 60 sec of side lunges	
11. 30 sec of plank	
12. 45 sec of burpees	
Repeat two or three times	

Cool Down and Stretch

Cool down and stretch protocols ensure that your heart rate lowers and you stretch your body in a manner that helps prevent injury and leads to faster recovery between workouts. These stretches can be undertaken between workouts to aide in faster recovery and reduce muscle soreness.

Refer to AwakenTheSexyWithin.com for your exercise demonstration and cool down and stretching program.

CAUTION: CONSULT A PHYSICIAN BEFORE USING THIS PROGRAM. STOP EXERCISING IF YOU FEEL PAIN, FAINT, DIZZY, OR SHORT OF BREATH.

Workout 44: Boxing Body Tone 2

Warm-up

Your 5-minute warm-up could be as simple as walking around the block, riding a stationary bike, doing 5 minutes of vigorous housework, etc. The important point is to ensure you are appropriately warmed up before performing any of the exercises.

Workout

This is a fantastic body-weighted workout, incorporating the fun principles and techniques of boxing. You can do this workout by yourself, you could use a punching bag, or you could use a partner working with some boxing pads. Make sure you refer to AwakenTheSexyWithin.com for the instructions on how to perform each boxing punch. Keep in mind that it's the technique and speed that count with the boxing for fitness and not trying to hit as hard as you can. Please also watch our brief video demonstrating the boxing basics. Go to AwakenTheSexyWithin.com to download the tools and watch the technique video.

Round 1 30 sec to complete each round	Round 2 1 min to complete each round	Round 3 1 min to complete each round
10 push-ups (30 sec) ⇔ jab and cross (30 sec)	10 squats (30 sec) ⇔ knees (30 sec)	6 squat thrusts ⇔ 11 push-ups ⇔ 16 squats
12 push-ups (30 sec) ⇔ upper cuts (30 sec)	12 squats (30 sec) ⇔ knees (30 sec)	1 min freestyle boxing
14 push-ups (30 sec) ⇔ blocks (30 sec)	14 squats (30 sec) ⇔ knees (30 sec)	7 squat thrusts ⇔ 12 push-ups ⇔. 17 squats
16 push-ups (30 sec) ⇔ jab and cross (30 sec)	16 squats (30 sec) ⇔ knees (30 sec)	1 min freestyle boxing
18 push-ups (30 sec) ⇔ upper cuts (30 sec)	18 squats (30 sec) ⇔ knees (30 sec)	8 squat thrusts ⇔ 13 push-ups ⇔ 18 squats
20 push-ups (30 sec) ⇔ blocks (30 sec)	20 squats (30 sec) ⇔ knees (30 sec)	1 min freestyle boxing
1 min rest	*1 min rest*	*1 min rest*

Round 4 *1 min to complete each round*	Round 5 *20 sec on 10 sec rest*		
20 sit-ups ⇔ 10 fast rows on the resistance band	Skipping (20 sec) ⇔ 10 sec res		
20 sit-ups ⇔ 12 fast rows on the resistance band			
20 sit-ups ⇔ 14 fast rows on the resistance band			
20 sit-ups ⇔ 16 fast rows on the resistance band	*Repeat for eight rounds*		
20 sit-ups ⇔ 14 fast rows on the resistance band			
20 sit-ups ⇔ 12 fast rows on the resistance band			
20 sit-ups ⇔ 10 fast rows on the resistance band			
1 min rest			

Cool Down and Stretch

Cool down and stretch protocols ensure that your heart rate lowers and you stretch your body in a manner that helps prevent injury and leads to faster recovery between workouts. These stretches can be undertaken between workouts to aide in faster recovery and reduce muscle soreness.

Refer to AwakenTheSexyWithin.com for your exercise demonstration and cool down and stretching program.

CAUTION: CONSULT A PHYSICIAN BEFORE USING THIS PROGRAM. STOP EXERCISING IF YOU FEEL PAIN, FAINT, DIZZY, OR SHORT OF BREATH.

Workout 45: Circuit Intensity 2

Warm-up

Your 5-minute warm-up could be as simple as walking around the block, riding a stationary bike, doing 5 minutes of vigorous housework, etc. The important point is to ensure you are appropriately warmed up before performing any of the exercises.

Workout

This is a great workout for the entire body, with aspects of cardio built in. With round 2, if 10 minutes is too long for your AMRAP (as many rounds as possible), then shorten it appropriately to suit your level of fitness. Enjoy this session, and put your mind into the muscle you are working with every single rep.

Round 1	Round 2	Round 3	Round 4	Round 5
3 min of shadow boxing—jab and cross	Complete 15 min of AMRAP	1 min of donkey kicks (30 sec each leg)	1 min of star jumps	30 sec of sit-ups
1 min of push-ups	25 squats	1 min of fire hydrants (30 sec each leg)	1 min of climbers	30 sec of back extensions
30 sec of dumb-bell military press	20 thrusts	1 min of hip raises (30 sec each leg)	1 min of high knees	20 sec of side planks (do both sides)
30 sec of dumb-bell lateral raises	10 bent-over rows	*Repeat*	*Repeat x 2*	30 sec of bicycle kicks
20 sec of front dumbbell raises	5 lunges			30 sec of leg raises
20 sec of criss-cross front dumbbells	10 squats			
20 sec of dumb-bell upright rows	15 thrusts			30 sec of criss-cross scissors
20 sec of push-ups	25 bent-over rows			

Cool Down and Stretch

Cool down and stretch protocols ensure that your heart rate lowers and you stretch your body in a manner that helps prevent injury and leads to faster recovery between workouts. These stretches can be undertaken between workouts to aide in faster recovery and reduce muscle soreness.

Refer to AwakenTheSexyWithin.com for your exercise demonstration and cool down and stretching program.

CAUTION: CONSULT A PHYSICIAN BEFORE USING THIS PROGRAM. STOP EXERCISING IF YOU FEEL PAIN, FAINT, DIZZY, OR SHORT OF BREATH.

Workout 46: Pack of Cards 3

Warm-up

Your 5-minute warm-up could be as simple as walking around the block, riding a stationary bike, doing 5 minutes of vigorous housework, etc. The important point is to ensure you are appropriately warmed up before performing any of the exercises.

Workout

This workout involves doing a workout with a pack of normal playing cards. Each suit of card is allocated an exercise, and you perform the number of repetitions on the card. Shuffle the deck of cards before you start. When a joker comes up, that's time to have a rest for up to 2 minutes. This is a fun workout and hard!

Exercise Description	
Hearts	Squats
Spades	Back extensions
Clubs	Push-ups
Diamonds	Jackknives or sit-ups
Aces	20 sec of squat jumps, 20 sec of power jacks, 20 sec of jumping jacks **(Repeat for 2 to 3 rounds per each Ace)**
Kings	60 sec of wall squats
Queens	60 sec of biceps curls
Jacks	60 sec of dips

Cool Down and Stretch

Cool down and stretch protocols ensure that your heart rate lowers and you stretch your body in a manner that helps prevent injury and leads to faster recovery between workouts. These stretches can be undertaken between workouts to aide in faster recovery and reduce muscle soreness.

Refer to AwakenTheSexyWithin.com for your exercise demonstration and cool down and stretching program.

CAUTION: CONSULT A PHYSICIAN BEFORE USING THIS PROGRAM. STOP EXERCISING IF YOU FEEL PAIN, FAINT, DIZZY, OR SHORT OF BREATH.

Workout 47: Three to Thrive

Warm-up

Your 5-minute warm-up could be as simple as walking around the block, riding a stationary bike, doing 5 minutes of vigorous housework, etc. The important point is to ensure you are appropriately warmed up before performing any of the exercises.

Workout

This is a great workout and can be performed with body-weighted exercises or kettlebells, resistance bands, dumbbells, or a combination. This workout is based on three rounds of timed duration. I have also provided several alternate exercises for you to select from. Make sure you don't always choose the easier option! If you want to make this workout more intense, once you finish all the exercises in round 3, repeat the workout from the beginning.

Round 1	Round 2	Round 3
60 sec of push-ups or hip thrust	60 sec of KB squats	60 sec of back extensions
30 sec of KB military press or hip raises	30 sec of lunges	30 sec of KB bent-over row or jumping jacks
30 sec of DB lat raises or hip raises	30 sec of squat jumps	30 sec of KB one-arm row or hips raises
30 sec of DB front raises or back extensions	30 sec of KB sumo squats	30 sec of kb one-arm row or hips raises
30 sec of DB criss-cross or KB sumo squats	30 sec of hip thrust	30 sec of RB biceps curls or squat jumps
30 sec of KB upright row or squat jumps	30 sec of calf raises	30 sec of dips or KB sumo squats
30 sec of push-ups or hip thrust	30 sec of KB squats	30 sec of back extensions
1 min rest	*1 min rest*	*1 min rest*
30 sec of heel touches 30 sec of leg raises 30 sec of plank 30 sec of sit-ups or crunch	30 sec of heel touches 30 sec of leg raises 30 sec of plank 30 sec of sit-ups or crunch	30 sec of heel touches 30 sec of leg raises 30 sec of plank 30 sec of sit-ups or crunch

Cool Down and Stretch

Cool down and stretch protocols ensure that your heart rate lowers and you stretch your body in a manner that helps prevent injury and leads to faster recovery between workouts. These stretches can be undertaken between workouts to aide in faster recovery and reduce muscle soreness.

Refer to AwakenTheSexyWithin.com for your exercise demonstration and cool down and stretching program.

CAUTION: CONSULT A PHYSICIAN BEFORE USING THIS PROGRAM. STOP EXERCISING IF YOU FEEL PAIN, FAINT, DIZZY, OR SHORT OF BREATH.

Workout 48: Let's Work It

Warm-up

Your 5-minute warm-up could be as simple as walking around the block, riding a stationary bike, doing 5 minutes of vigorous housework, etc. The important point is to ensure you are appropriately warmed up before performing any of the exercises.

Workout

The focus of this workout is legs, arms, abdominal muscles, and cardio. Each round is timed for either 30 or 45 seconds, with minimal rest in between sets. You can adjust the intensity of each exercise by performing more or fewer repetitions for each.

Round 1 45 sec for each exercise	Round 2 45 sec for each exercise	Round 3 45 sec for each exercise	Round 4 45 sec for each exercise	Round 5 45 sec for each exercise
1. Squat (15 sec to transition)	1. Burpees (15 sec to transition)	1. 10 biceps curls => 10 dips	1. RB boxing—jab and cross	1. Bicycle abs
2. Squat hold (15 sec to transition)	2. Climbers (15 sec to transition)	2. 12 biceps curls => 12 dips	2. RB boxing—upper cuts	2. Leg raises
3. Step-ups (15 sec to transition)	3. Thrusts (15 sec to transition)	3. 14 biceps curls => 14 dips	3. RB boxing—rips	3. Russian twists
4. Squat thrusts (15 sec to transition)	4. Skipping (15 sec to transition)	4. 12 biceps curls => 12 dips	4. RB boxing—jab and cross	4. Side plank (left)
5. Lunges (15 sec to transition)	5. Jumping jacks (15 sec to transition)	5. 10 biceps curls => 10 dips	5. RB boxing—upper cuts	5. Side plank (right)
Repeat x 2 or 3	*Repeat x 2 or 3*		6. RB boxing—rips	
1 min rest	*1 min rest*	*1 min rest*	*1 min rest and repeat*	*Cool down and stretch*

Cool Down and Stretch

Cool down and stretch protocols ensure that your heart rate lowers and you stretch your body in a manner that helps prevent injury and leads to faster recovery between workouts. These stretches can be undertaken between workouts to aide in faster recovery and reduce muscle soreness.

Refer to AwakenTheSexyWithin.com for your exercise demonstration and cool down and stretching program.

CAUTION: CONSULT A PHYSICIAN BEFORE USING THIS PROGRAM. STOP EXERCISING IF YOU FEEL PAIN, FAINT, DIZZY, OR SHORT OF BREATH.

Workout 49: Four Rounds to Hell 3

Warm-up

Your 5-minute warm-up could be as simple as walking around the block, riding a stationary bike, doing 5 minutes of vigorous housework, etc. The important point is to ensure you are appropriately warmed up before performing any of the exercises.

Workout

This workout involves overloading the muscles, as well as taxing the aerobic system. It's a great workout to perform with a buddy but still possible by yourself. Refer to AwakenTheSexyWithin.com and our video at AwakenTheSexyWithin. com for boxing techniques, how to perform with a partner and without. Don't forget: Have fun! This is a tough workout, but you'll feel amazing by the end!

Round 1	Round 2	Round 3	Round 4
45 sec of butt kicks	10 burpees	10 bent-over rows	60 sec of 10 jab and cross => 3 push-ups
45 sec of sumo squats	10 push-ups	10 frog squat jumps	60 sec of 4 knees => 4 squat jumps
45 sec of star jumps	*Repeat for 3 rounds*	*Repeat for 3 rounds*	60 sec of 10 jab and cross with sit-ups
Repeat for 3 rounds	30 burpees	30 bent-over rows	
30 sec plank	30 push-ups	30 frog squat jumps	20 sec of jab and cross 20 sec of upper cut 20 sec of blocks
30 sec jackknives	*Rest 30 sec*	*Rest 30 sec*	
30 sec heel touches	20 sec climbers		
30 sec double crunches	20 sec squat jumps		
30 sec knees in and out	20 sec push-ups	*1min rest*	
30 sec side-to-side abs	20 sec jumping jacks		
Repeat for 2 rounds	*Repeat for 3 rounds*		*Repeat*
1 min rest	*1 min rest*		

Cool Down and Stretch

Cool down and stretch protocols ensure that your heart rate lowers and you stretch your body in a manner that helps prevent injury and leads to faster recovery between workouts. These stretches can be undertaken between workouts to aide in faster recovery and reduce muscle soreness.

Refer to AwakenTheSexyWithin.com for your exercise demonstration and cool down and stretching program.

CAUTION: CONSULT A PHYSICIAN BEFORE USING THIS PROGRAM. STOP EXERCISING IF YOU FEEL PAIN, FAINT, DIZZY, OR SHORT OF BREATH.

Workout 50: Sneaky

Warm-up

Your 5-minute warm-up could be as simple as walking around the block, riding a stationary bike, doing 5 minutes of vigorous housework, etc. The important point is to ensure you are appropriately warmed up before performing any of the exercises.

Workout

I call this workout "sneaky" because it really does sneak up on you. It doesn't seem difficult to start with but slowly grabs hold of you. It's a fantastic workout; be sure to refer to AwakenTheSexyWithin.com to ensure your technique is current for this workout.

Round 1	Round 2	Round 3	Round 4
10 squat to stand	8 bent-over rows	8 each side split squats	8 each side single leg hip thrust
10 alternating lunges	10 each side kneeling hip flexor	12 leg raises to 90 degrees	20 sec sumo squat stretch
10 alternating lateral lunges		30 sec each side plank (right and left)	10 goblet squat
10 stationery Spider-man	*Repeat for a total of 3 sets*		
10 scapular push-ups		*Repeat for a total of 3 sets*	*Repeat for a total of 3 sets*

Cool Down and Stretch

Cool down and stretch protocols ensure that your heart rate lowers and you stretch your body in a manner that helps prevent injury and leads to faster recovery between workouts. These stretches can be undertaken between workouts to aide in faster recovery and reduce muscle soreness.

Refer to AwakenTheSexyWithin.com for your exercise demonstration and cool down and stretching program.

CAUTION: CONSULT A PHYSICIAN BEFORE USING THIS PROGRAM. STOP EXERCISING IF YOU FEEL PAIN, FAINT, DIZZY, OR SHORT OF BREATH.

Workout 51: Magnificent Seven

Warm-up

Your 5-minute warm-up could be as simple as walking around the block, riding a stationary bike, doing 5 minutes of vigorous housework, etc. The important point is to ensure you are appropriately warmed up before performing any of the exercises.

Workout

This workout works around the theme of seven. Complete this workout in your fastest possible time, making sure that you take note of how many rounds you have completed (because you can lose count easily). Record your time, and aim to beat it next time you complete this workout. Make sure you have a stopwatch for this workout.

If you are outside, set up some cone markers for 7 sprints at 20 yards for beginners, 25 yards for intermediate, and 30 yards for advanced (up and back is 2 sprints).

Exercise Description
1. 70 skipping revolutions (jumping jacks or side-to-side steps for alternatives)
2. 7 burpees (squat jumps or squats for those that can't do burpees, but they must do 2 for every 1 burpee)
3. 7 push-ups chest to the floor
4. 7 squats with 20 pounds of weight
5. 7 resistance band rows with a 2-sec hold
6. 7 full sit-ups (7 crunches with a 2-sec hold if you can't do sit-ups)
7. Super-fast jab and cross shadow boxing (140 beginner, 175 for intermediate, 210 for advanced)
1 min rest between each of the seven rounds

Cool Down and Stretch

Cool down and stretch protocols ensure that your heart rate lowers and you stretch your body in a manner that helps prevent injury and leads to faster recovery between workouts. These stretches can be undertaken between workouts to aide in faster recovery and reduce muscle soreness.

Refer to AwakenTheSexyWithin.com for your exercise demonstration and cool down and stretching program.

CAUTION: CONSULT A PHYSICIAN BEFORE USING THIS PROGRAM. STOP EXERCISING IF YOU FEEL PAIN, FAINT, DIZZY, OR SHORT OF BREATH.

Workout 52: Pyramids in Japan

Warm-up
Your 5-minute warm-up could be as simple as walking around the block, riding a stationary bike, doing 5 minutes of vigorous housework, etc. The important point is to ensure you are appropriately warmed up before performing any of the exercises.

Workout
This aimed at taxing the aerobic system as well as the anaerobic system. Each segment runs for exactly 1 minute. Each person has 60 seconds to perform each of the required 20 exercises. If they finish early, they rest for the remaining time. If someone fails to complete all the requirements within the timeframe, they must sit out the next minute and recover. They can then join in the next round.

Round 1

Exercise Description	Exercise Description
30 skips + 1 bent-over rows	30 skips + 11 bent-over rows
30 skips + 2 bent-over rows	30 skips + 12 bent-over rows
30 skips + 3 bent-over rows	30 skips + 13 bent-over rows
30 skips + 4 bent-over rows	30 skips + 14 bent-over rows
30 skips + 5 bent-over rows	30 skips + 15 bent-over rows
30 skips + 6 bent-over rows	30 skips + 16 bent-over rows
30 skips + 7 bent-over rows	30 skips + 17 bent-over rows
30 skips + 8 bent-over rows	30 skips + 18 bent-over rows
30 skips + 9 bent-over rows	30 skips + 19 bent-over rows
30 skips + 10 bent-over rows	30 skips + 20 bent-over rows

Round 2
The Tabata protocol was invented by a Japanese exercise scientist Dr. Izumi Tabata. This style of short, intense interval training has shown to have a dramatic improvement on anaerobic capacity and oxygen uptake. The aim of this work out is 20 seconds of all-out effort, followed by 10 seconds of rest => repeated eight times, for a total of 4 minutes. Allow 2 minutes rest between each set.

Exercise Description
1. Kettlebell sumo squat ⇔ upright rows (alternate each 20 sec)
2. Squat jumps ⇔ climbers (alternate each 20 sec)
3. Kettlebell swings
4. On the spot sprint or high knees
5. Surrenders

Round 3

Exercise Description
1. 30 sec of windshield wipers
2. 30 sec of Russian twists
3. 30 sec of side-to-side abs
4. 30 sec of plank with toe taps

Cool Down and Stretch

Cool down and stretch protocols ensure that your heart rate lowers and you stretch your body in a manner that helps prevent injury and leads to faster recovery between workouts. These stretches can be undertaken between workouts to aide in faster recovery and reduce muscle soreness.

Refer to AwakenTheSexyWithin.com for your exercise demonstration and cool down and stretching program.

CAUTION: CONSULT A PHYSICIAN BEFORE USING THIS PROGRAM. STOP EXERCISING IF YOU FEEL PAIN, FAINT, DIZZY, OR SHORT OF BREATH.

SUCCESS STORY:
Kez Shiels, 27 years old

Kez lost 46 pounds (24.3% weight loss), reduced her body fat by 19.5%, and lost a total of 39 inches from her chest, waist, hips, arms, and thighs.

"People that haven't seen me for a while can't believe just how much I've changed my body and want to know what I'm doing and how! I love my training, have now taken up some bike riding, and recently had my cholesterol levels tested, and it's the lowest it's ever been!"

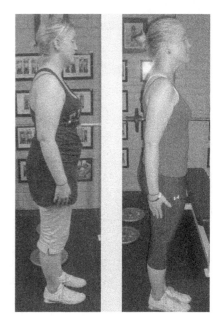

CHAPTER 7

Maintaining Your Sexiness

e careful what you wish for. There's a wonderful scene from the movie classic *Chariots of Fire*. For those of you that don't know the movie, it follows the true-life story of two runners, Eric Liddell and Harold Abrahams, who qualify to compete at the 1924 Olympic Games, in Paris. It's a very compelling movie. After a harrowing road to the Olympics, Harold wins the 100-meter race. While everyone around him celebrates, he is silent and overwhelmed by the enormity of what he has just accomplished. He had worked so hard, for so long, to achieve Olympic Gold but didn't know what he would do when he won.

If you adhere to the programming in *Awaken the Sexy within*, you *will* get to the body you desire. It's not a question of *if* but rather a question of *when*. The danger I see with most clients is the closer they get to their goals, the more complacent they may get. Progress can stop or regress. That's not an outcome we want for you. We must always be making progress; otherwise, we will not be fulfilled. Don't forget that achieving and maintaining your sexiness is a life-long journey. We should be looking to make improvements every day.

The goal of this chapter is to help you prepare for the day you hit your goals. I don't want you to be overwhelmed by the enormity of what you've accomplished, and I don't want to see your hard-won results slip away. So even though you are

219

still likely at the beginning of your journey, I'd like you to picture a future in which you've accomplished all the goals you've made for yourself so far.

Your Sexiness Has Been Awakened!

Let's fast-forward to the day that you realize you have completely awoken the sexy version of yourself and achieved the body you desire. *Congratulations! You are completely awesome!*

What an amazing achievement. Look back on the photos you took at the very beginning of the journey, and reconnect with *why* you set out to change your body in the first place. Go back to the mirror, and ask yourself if you feel more comfortable in your own skin now than you did when you took those original photos. Have you begun to appreciate your body and all it can do more?

If so, the first thing to do is celebrate, and how you celebrate is important. In Western culture, a celebration conjures up images of food, alcohol, and lots of it! I am suggesting that you celebrate your success in a way that empowers you, not that partially undoes some of your hard work.

Here's some examples of how you can celebrate:

- Acknowledge to yourself what an incredible person you are and how proud you are. Recognize that you have undertaken a lot of hard work and are now enjoying the fruits of your labor. You may have had to battle those negative voices to get here. So stand up. Be proud. Love yourself! Spoil yourself with a small gift. If you've been wanting a new pair of headphones to work out with, this could be the time to get them for yourself. Keep the gift related to your workout routine if possible. Try a new restaurant, but keep it healthy. Perhaps you could step outside your comfort zone and find a delicious vegetarian or vegan restaurant.
- Throw a healthy celebration dinner party for some close friends or family that have supported you on your journey.
- Invest in a self-improvement program or a book in another area of interest to help take your life to a new level.
- Go to a concert of your favorite artist.
- Get away. Head to the spa, go on a weekend trip, or just go on a nice hike. Do something you love that's out of your ordinary routine.

- Treat yourself to a night at the movies.
- Go to the theatre to see a new show.
- Take some time out for yourself to learn a new hobby.
- Anything else that you can think of that will make you feel like you are celebrating in an empowering manner.

The next step is to set some new goals. I work with clients to create new goals before they reach their current targets. The importance of this is to ensure you are always aiming for a target that's slightly ahead of you. That is how you keep moving forward.

The next set of tasks for you is only to be completed when you are getting close to the goals you set in chapter 1, and you'll follow the same process. Be patient, be consistent, and complete all the other tasks before you complete this one. Mark it in your calendar now to come back to this chapter so that you don't forget.

Determining your new goals once you are close to achieving your existing ones can be challenging. The competitive athlete always has that next competition coming up, which creates focus and drive toward those events. But what if you don't have competitions or events to plan for? Let me give you some examples of goals that you can set for yourself:

- Complete a 3-mile, 6-mile, or half-marathon run for fun. There are dozens of these formally organized around the world.
- Join a running group in your town.
- Train for a triathlon.
- Go on a challenging hike.
- Take up cycling.
- Compete in an ultramarathon event.
- Train to hike a mountain.
- Use your fitness assessment to set new performance goals.
- Sign up for a volleyball, softball, or other sports league with friends.
- Learn to rock climb.
- Take up dancing.
- Take up swimming or rowing.
- Learn to surf.
- Take a snow skiing lesson.

- Check out my Road to 600 project, which I undertook on Facebook and Instagram

ACTION 40: DEFINING YOUR NEXT-LEVEL GOALS

Taking the ideas above into consideration, write down your next-level goals, which will drive you beyond your initial body transformation and into a new level of thinking of what is possible for you.

Challenge yourself. What goals do you have for yourself over the next 12 months?

1 Year Health and Fitness Goals

Quarterly Goals
Qtr. 1. January to March
Qtr. 2. April to June
Qtr. 3. July to September
Qtr. 4. October to December

DO NOT MOVE ON TO THE NEXT CHAPTER UNTIL YOU HAVE COMPLETED EVERY ACTION ITEM ABOVE. NO EXCUSES!

Summary

- It's not a question of *if* but, rather, a question of *when* you will awaken the sexy within.
- It's important to celebrate your success along the way but also to ensure you have awoken your sexy within.
- Don't become complacent when you are close to achieving your ultimate sexy body.
- Set new challenging goals in areas that improve and motivate you to take your new body to even greater heights.

CHAPTER 8

What's Next?

C ongratulations on getting to our final chapter in this amazing transformation we have taken together. If you have completed all 40 of the
action tasks I've outlined, then I know you will now be living your life
on a new level. You will have a new empowered mindset. You will have already
created changes necessary to transform your body. You will have a hunger to create
a better version of yourself on a continuous basis.

You have all the tools. Now, it's about consistency and keeping on adhering
to the principles outlined in the preceding eight chapters.

If you *haven't* completed every single action task in this book, you will be missing an opportunity to reach your maximum potential. Please go back and complete every action task you skipped. They have been proven repeatedly to work.

At this point, you may well be asking, "What's next? What do I do now?"

When I'm working with clients that either get very close to their goals or
have achieved them, I find that plateaus, or even regression, can occur. There
can be multiple reasons for this, but I believe complacency is the main reason.
Justifying to ourselves that close enough is good enough. Not stretching ourselves to reach another level because we've done a good job to get where we
are now. We're doing better than most, so it's okay to stop striving for new
goals now.

I network with people around the world, and there are many traits that cross all human characteristics and behaviors, irrespective of the country they live, their religion, sex, relationship status, skin color, employment status, age, or fitness level. The bottom line is that most people on this planet we call Earth will go to the grave leaving their dreams unfulfilled. Not achieving the goals that they once had. Leaving books unwritten. Products uncreated. Relationships less rich and meaningful. Visions unseen. Potential untapped. We don't push ourselves hard enough. We don't take massive action to shift our thinking and lives to a level we would consider "outstanding." We become complacent in achieving "something" but what we are truly capable of is much deeper and meaningful. The question is *How do we tap into that energy that moves us into the unknown territory of greatness?*

My favorite challenge for every person that achieves their initial health and fitness goals is to find a way to think beyond themselves and contribute to others. This is one of life's most beautiful gifts. I feel that we humans were created to help coach each other to a greater level of living. It is like fuel for our souls. Once we start, it fills us up and makes us want to give more. It's why we say to our children that it is better to give presents at Christmas time rather than receive them. And one day, they'll believe us.

When I was working as an auditor, I was part of a team that discovered over $110 million in savings for a company. It was a huge amount, and it felt great to support a client like that. But that feeling paled in comparison to helping my first client, Stephen, lose 22 pounds (10 kilograms) in 6 weeks. I can still remember the smile on his face at weigh-in. I saw how my actions could have a real impact on someone's life, and it felt incredible. So incredible that I dedicated my life to it.

And now that I get paid for it, I look for additional ways to contribute to people's lives. I believe there is a deeper meaning to our life when we don't expect anything in return—when we give our time to a worthy cause just because it is the right thing to do. You've raised yourself to a higher level of living, of health, of fitness, and of purpose in your life. It's now time to lean down, put out your hand, and pull someone else up to where you are. It's an incredible source of food for the soul.

I love my job, and I am fortunate to make a successful income from my business. This success enables me to help others in a variety of ways in my local community. For instance, I created several free health and fitness programs as my way of giving back. These include

- The Kids Munch It program (www.KidsMunchIt.com.au) is a free nutrition program that I deliver to children from preschool to high school in our local shire.
- Family Food Rescue (www.FamilyFoodRescue.com.au) is a free program designed to work with individual families requiring a health and fitness overhaul. This program focuses on the adults and children to overhaul their mindsets, bodies, and nutrition through education, inspiration, and empowerment. From workouts, cooking classes, pantry, and fridge and freezer makeovers to transformational vocabulary, this program leaves no stone unturned.
- Local charitable causes. At the time of writing *Awaken the Sexy within*, our business has donated more than $250,000 of services within our community to worthy causes.

The mindset behind developing all these programs has been to follow my heart and be innovative in the way I can use my skills and passion to positively affect people's lives. The more money I make through my businesses, the greater the opportunity I have to help others.

That is a beautiful gift, and I am so gracious to be able to contribute in the way that I do.

Perhaps you already have some ideas about how you can give beyond yourself. Jot some of those thoughts down right now before you lose them. We are going to do an exercise very shortly to take these thoughts to the next level.

Tony Robbins has had a tremendously powerful impact on my life by helping me become more passionate, driven, spiritual, and focused about what is important in my life. Tony talks about the six human needs. He discusses them in the context of them not being wants but needs that every human has. For completeness, the first four are *significance, certainty, variety,* and *love and connection.* Tony suggests that we all find a way to meet these needs in one way or another. Even if they are disempowering methods, we still find a way of meeting them. For instance, a gang member can meet their need for significance using violence. You can meet these first four needs and still not feel complete. Tony says it is the last two needs that enable us to live an abundant, complete and fulfilled life. The final two human needs are *growth* and *contribution*. By completing the 40 tasks already outlined in this book, you will have already experienced an incredible level of growth and transformation. For us to be happy and fulfilled we *must* grow. You must always maintain a high standard for yourself and grow continuously. Look at the most successful people in the world, and you will find that they have a focus on their personal growth.

It's now time to focus on contribution. Studies have shown that happier people give more and that giving makes people happier. This can result in a continuous loop of giving making you happy, making others happier, making you even happier, resulting in you giving more to make even more people happier!

You may already have ideas as to how you would like to contribute to others, but if you don't, here are 20 ways to volunteer your time that may ignite a fire within you:

1. Volunteer at a local school. This could involve spending time reading, tutoring, helping in the kitchens, working in the garden, etc.
2. Find local charities you are passionate about and reach out to them to learn about volunteer opportunities.
3. Volunteer at retirement facilities. Many residents do not receive regular visitors and appreciate someone to talk to and share life's stories.
4. The Men's Shed project is a popular Australian initiative that has had tremendous success among retired men wanting to share their handyman and craft skills with others. Similar projects are available around the world that work specifically with retired men.
5. Local community gardens. If you're a green thumb, or want to become one, this is a great option to mix with locals passionate about everything that grows.
6. Local sports clubs are in constant need of volunteers to help them support their members excel in the activities they love. Opportunities include coaching, first aid, mentoring, fitness training, massage therapy, nutrition support and guidance, supervision, working in the canteen, fundraising—you name it, they will appreciate the help.

7. Helping the homeless. Homelessness is a worldwide problem and thankfully there are many organizations working hard to serve those in need. Find one near you and get involved. It could involve working in one of their thrift shops, fundraising, requesting donations of clothes and blankets, or serving meals.

8. Become involved on a community board. I've sat on community boards before, and it can be a very fulfilling role to know that you are having a positive impact in your community.

9. Volunteer at your local library, museum, art gallery, national trust property, zoo, aquarium, etc. These organizations thrive from the time that volunteers provide for a range of roles in administration, cleaning, maintenance, and guiding tours. Enthusiasm, passion, patience, and flexibility are usually the only requirements to get involved.

10. Organize a local walking group among your neighbors. Not only will you get to know your neighbors, but it also increases your sense of personal security and builds a stronger sense of community.

11. Volunteering at a hospital is an option for some hospitals. We have very strict privacy laws in Australia, so the range of functions you perform can be limited, but there may be options available in administration, working in the kitchens, sitting with patients, etc.

12. Telephone contact center help desks are a great way to volunteer your time if you are passionate about helping those in need. Volunteer for a veteran help line or a suicide prevention help line.

13. You could knit for the needy locally or in other countries.

14. Create your own podcast series, blog, vlog, or Facebook page designed to help others improve their lives.

15. Become a St. John Ambulance or Red Cross volunteer, and improve your first-aid skills in the process. Often underrated, but both organizations will be very busy in your community every single week. I was a member of St. John Ambulance for many years and found it incredibly rewarding. You meet some amazing people.

16. Work for Rotary Club, Lions Club, or other organizations that serve your community and abroad.

17. Bake some healthy muffins, and introduce yourself to your new neighbors. It's a great icebreaker and a lovely way to start off your relationship with them. Trust me, people don't do these types of things anymore, so make a difference on your street by stepping up to give back!

18. Next time you approach a homeless person, and they ask you for some loose change, why not give them $20 instead? Take out your wallet, hand over the money, and tell them that you believe in them and that things can turn around for them.

19. Mow your neighbor's front lawn. I figure if you've got the lawn mower out and you've mown your grass, it doesn't take too much effort to spend 5 minutes cutting your neighbor's. Where I live, that's all it takes. It's just a nice thing to do, expecting nothing in return.

20. Provide a copy of *Awaken the Sexy within* to someone who is important to you. Talk to them about the impact that this has had on your transformation and how it can help them. Be an inspiration and a source of everything that is beautiful and wonderful about health and fitness. Keep the conversations going with those that require more support, and use the action steps you have learned here to shift their thinking to a more resourceful place of action.

Remember, what you put out will come back to you tenfold in ways that you may never expect. You contribute to others not because you know it will come back but because it makes you feel happier about the person you are.

ACTION 41: DEFINING CONTRIBUTION BEYOND YOURSELF

Take 5 minutes to write down all the ways in which you can contribute beyond yourself. Select areas that you are deeply passionate about, and use my list of 20 above to get your creative juices flowing.

_____

_____

_____

_____

_____

_____

_____

_____

ACTION 42: DEFINING THE MEANING OF YOUR CONTRIBUTION

Write down the powerful emotions you will feel once you start contributing in these areas. What will that mean to you? What will it bring into your life? Be sure to use emotive and descriptive language that is meaningful to you.

_____

_____

_____

_____

_____

_____

_____

ACTION 43: NOW ACT!

Write down your best idea from action task 41, where you believe you can passionately contribute to others without expecting anything in return. Write down specifically the action you will take in the next 24 hours to move yourself at least one step closer to achieving your outcome of contributing to others. Then go out and do it!

_____

_____

_____

_____

_____

_____

_____

Knowing that you have contributed your time with the expectation of receiving no financial reward is a beautiful opportunity for you to grow in ways you never thought possible. My children often ask me if I'd like to be famous one day, and I tell them I wouldn't like the loss of privacy, but I would love to be in a position where I could help more people. Sometimes, just the presence of someone in a room can make you feel more alive, vibrant, and driven to be a better version of yourself. Imagine if that was you. You don't have to be famous to make a difference in a truly meaningful way in this world we live. All that is stopping you right now is your mindset.

Be open to the idea of you contributing to others, and it will reveal another side of you that you didn't know existed. It's an exciting journey that you'll wish you had begun a long time ago.

DO NOT MOVE ON TO THE NEXT CHAPTER UNTIL YOU HAVE COMPLETED EVERY ACTION ITEM ABOVE. NO EXCUSES!

Summary

- One of life's greatest gifts is to contribute beyond ourselves to help others.
- Contributing to others is food for the soul.
- Contribution must be made with sincerity, integrity, enthusiasm, and passion to be meaningful in your life.
- You must not expect anything in return for your contribution to others.
- Use the examples in this chapter to help you identify ways in which you can contribute to others.
- What you put out will come back to you tenfold in a way that you may never expect.
- The more you contribute to others, the more fulfilled you will feel, and the more you will want to give.

SUCCESS STORY:
Lauren Stapleton, 35 years old

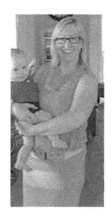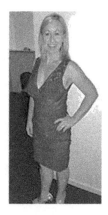

Lauren has now lost over 22 pounds of body fat and a total of 18 inches off her waist, chest, hips, arms, and legs to completely transform herself after her first baby. She is now in better shape than her prebaby body.

"I had been looking for ways to shift the 66 pounds I had put on with my first baby. By August of the same year, I had hit a standstill with my weight loss. I had seen other people have heaps of success with Robb's program, so I thought, Why not?! I have consistently stuck to the program, and I am now back to my prebaby weight and feel great. I still want to lose 10 pounds

more and to tone up further, just so I can once again be my prewedding weight. I've started running again, with the aim of running my first 8-mile event. Overall, I feel great. I highly recommend trying Robb's program if you are struggling to achieve your weight-loss goals."

CONCLUSION

Final Thoughts

I'd like to take this opportunity to thank you for investing the time, money, and resources in *Awaken the Sexy within*, but most of all, in yourself. All too often, we humans find a way to not prioritize our health, our fitness, and our wellness and specifically set aside time to grow ourselves and contribute to others. In these final words, you may feel that this is the end of a beautiful journey. In many ways, this is just the beginning. I recommend that you read this book multiple times and complete the action tasks each time. In 6 months, a year, 2 years, or 5 years, you will be in a different place in your life, and each step will have different meaning to you. Each time you act, you will obtain and different outcome. My vision for you is that you *never* stop growing and that you never lose the hunger to make yourself and your health, mind, and body better than you were the day before.

I am very proud to deliver you my first book, *Awaken the Sexy within*. I trust that you have enjoyed reading it and are now a walking success story. Congratulations! The exciting news is that I have three other books in my *Sexy* series underway, so be sure to take up the bonuses below to stay fully up to date with their launch dates.

Life is beautiful, and living it with vital health and abundant energy is the ultimate gift we should all give to ourselves. My team and I would love to hear from you, so please share your success stories with us on our social media platforms. I hope to meet you face to face one day so that we can celebrate your success together.

Make today count! Make tomorrow count! Make the rest of your life count!

Sexy Bonuses!

Congratulations on getting to this page because I know you will have implemented all the steps I've asked you to and are getting amazing results. Contained in this chapter are your FREE bonus gifts that you receive by purchasing *Awaken the Sexy within*. These bonuses are valued at $498 and have been personally handpicked by me to support you in furthering your body transformation.

Please take advantage of these gifts:

Bonus 1: One FREE 45-minute body transformation coaching session with me personally. This session can be conducted in person or via phone, Skype, Zoom, WhatsApp, etc. You can obtain your FREE session by registering at www. StudiozPT.com.au and providing the code ATSW45.

Bonus 2: Access to six FREE health and fitness reports. You can download the reports by visiting www.StudiozPT.com.au.

Bonus 3: FREE subscription to our monthly newsletter. By registering for any of our free reports or coaching sessions, you will automatically become sub-scribed to our monthly newsletter.

Bonus 4: If you are local to one of our boot camp programs, you can register for 4 weeks FREE of our Pakenham Boot Camps for Women program. You can register at www.PakenhamBootCampsForWomen.com.au.

Bonus 5: You can now get 365 days of coaching, motivation, life and business lessons, as well as behind-the-scenes access to by subscribing to my FREE podcast by visiting www.RobbEvans365.com or downloading from any of the popular platforms, including iTunes, Spotify, Amazon Music, and Google Podcast.

Bonus 6: If you would like to have your own individually tailored meal plan created by my team, you can take advantage of our special offer by contacting us via www.StudiozPT.com.au and providing the code ATSW45.

About The Author

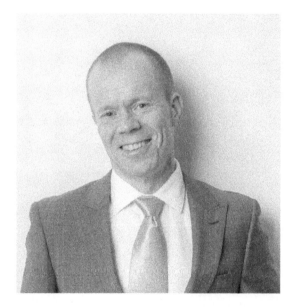

As a health services professional with over 30 years of experience in the field, Robb Evans is recognized and trusted for his expertise in the health and fitness area. He is the owner of a successful health, fitness, and nutrition business and specializes in coaching people to reach their fitness goals through creating new sustainable habits, proper nutrition, cardiovascular exercise, and effective resistance-training techniques. Robb prides himself on educating his clients so that they can live a fit and healthy lifestyle forever. He currently resides in Pakenham, Victoria, in Australia.

To find out more information about Robb,
check out the website www.AwakentheSexyWithin.com

CPSIA information can be obtained
at www.ICGtesting.com
Printed in the USA
LVHW091119230420
653674LV00022B/219